ASSESSMENT SKILLS LABORATORY MANUAL FOR

HEALTH
&
PHYSICAL ASSESSMENT
IN NURSING

ASSESSMENT SKILLS LABORATORY MANUAL FOR

HEALTH

&

PHYSICAL ASSESSMENT IN NURSING

Elizabeth Farren Corbin, Ph. D., FNP., RN
Professor of Nursing
Baylor University School of Nursing
Dallas, Texas

Donita D'Amico, MEd, RN
Associate Professor
William Paterson University
Wayne, New Jersey

Colleen Barbarito, EdD, RN
Assistant Professor
William Paterson University
Wayne, New Jersey

PEARSON

Prentice Hall

Upper Saddle River, New Jersey 07458

Publisher: Julie Levin Alexander
Publisher's Assistant: Regina Bruno
Editor-in-Chief: Maura Connor
Acquisitions Editor: Pamela Fuller
Associate Editor: Michael Giacobbe
Editorial Assistant: Melisa Baez
Director of Manufacturing and Production: Bruce Johnson
Managing Production Editor: Patrick Walsh
Production Liaison: Cathy O'Connell
Production Editor: Emily Bush, Carlisle Publishing Services
Manufacturing Manager: Ilene Sanford
Manufacturing Buyer: Pat Brown
Design Director: Maria Guglielmo
Director of Marketing: Karen Allman
Senior Marketing Manager: Francisco Del Castillo
Marketing Coordinator: Michael Sirinides
Marketing Assistant: Patricia Linard
Media Editor: John Jordan
Media Production Manager: Amy Peltier
Media Project Manager: Tina Rudowski
Composition: Carlisle Publishing Services
Printer/Binder: Command Web
Cover Printer: Phoenix Color
Cover Photo: Courtesy of Digital Vision/Getty Images, Inc.

Notice: Care has been taken to confirm the accuracy of information presented in this book. The authors, editors, and publisher, however, cannot accept any responsibility for errors or omissions or for consequences from application of the information in this book and make no warranty, express or implied, with respect to its contents.

The authors and publisher have exerted every effort to ensure that drug selections and dosages set forth in this text are in accord with current recommendations and practice at time of publication. However, in view of ongoing research, changes in government regulations, and the constant flow of information relating to drug therapy and drug reactions, the reader is urged to check the package inserts of all drugs for any change in indications of dosage and for added warnings and precautions. This is particularly important when the recommended agent is a new and/or infrequently employed drug.

Pearson Prentice Hall™ is a trademark of Pearson Education, Inc.
Pearson® is a registered trademark of Pearson plc
Prentice Hall® is a registered trademark of Pearson Education, Inc.

Pearson Education Ltd.
Pearson Education Singapore, Pte. Ltd.
Pearson Education Canada, Ltd.
Pearson Education—Japan

Pearson Education Australia PTY, Limited
Pearson Education North Asia Ltd.
Pearson Educación de Mexico, S.A. de C.V.
Pearson Education Malaysia, Pte. Ltd
Pearson Education, Upper Saddle River, NJ

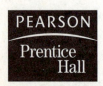

10 9 8 7 6 5 4 3 2
ISBN: 0-13-049477-1

Preface

Health assessment is the foundation for any and all nursing interventions. Of all healthcare providers, nurses approach the client in the most comprehensive and holistic manner, concerning themselves not just with disease process but with aspects of the client's life that maintain and enhance health and promote a fulfilling life. The **Assessment Skills Laboratory Manual** is designed to support and put into motion the principles of a thorough health and physical assessment, as set forth in **Health & Physical Assessment in Nursing,** by Donita D'Amico and Colleen Barbarito.

Initial chapters in both the text and the laboratory manual provide you with a comprehensive understanding of health assessment and health promotion and the variations that occur in each developmental stage. The book then acquaints you with the techniques, equipment, and tools used to perform and document a health and physical assessment. Chapters 11 through 24 take you systematically through all the body systems, and the final three chapters provide you with techniques needed to assess infants, children, older people, and pregnant women.

Each chapter in the laboratory manual corresponds to a chapter in the text and begins with an overview that summarizes the purpose of the chapter. A list of vocabulary is presented to prepare you to use the language of the particular area of assessment under consideration. You will want to familiarize yourself with the vocabulary as you prepare to carry out the assessment activities in each chapter. This will deepen your understanding of concepts and enable you to begin documenting your assessment findings professionally. In each chapter you will also find the following features that will call for you to enter actively into the assessment process:

- *Readings* and *media tools* remind you of the rich learning resources available to you through your textbook.
- *Labeling Exercises* present anatomical drawings or assessment tools, such as pain scales, that correspond to the subject of assessment in that chapter. This exercise is designed to help you succeed in actually performing assessment techniques.
- *Study Focus* questions direct your thinking not just to techniques of assessment but to the core reasons for assessments and their use in treating the client.
- *Review Questions* are presented in a variety of forms to help you prepare for testing and discussion of important aspects of each specific assessment focus.
- *Case Studies* illustrate the use of assessment techniques and findings in the care of real clients. Using these studies as discussions with classmates and instructors will enlarge your understanding of the application of assessment skills and the critical thinking used in planning appropriate care.
- *Clinical Activities* offer you the opportunity to perform assessment skills and provide you with additional advice on their use.

Throughout the laboratory manual you are encouraged to discuss and share thoughts and information with your peers, your preceptors, and especially your instructors. Excellent health and physical assessment is a skill that can be perfected and an art that will continue to grow as you nurture it. Nursing has a unique and privileged position in helping clients protect and improve their health from wherever they are on the continuum of health when they come under our care. It is my hope that this little book will be a help to you in beginning your skills of health and physical assessment. May the Nightingale force be with you!

Elizabeth Farren Corbin, Ph. D., FNP, RN
Professor of Nursing
Baylor University School of Nursing

Contents

Health Assessment

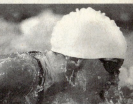

OVERVIEW

Chapter 1 introduces you to health assessment as a crucial nursing responsibility and to the style and presentation of the *Health & Physical Assessment in Nursing* textbook. This chapter presents definitions of health, a brief discussion of the focus of the healthcare system, the nursing process, and the cognitive skill of critical thinking.

The systematic collection of data required for health assessment is outlined, as are techniques for data collection, organization, and documentation. Clinical thinking is introduced in the discussion of interpretation of findings and the development of nursing plans to address client problems and needs. This chapter forms the foundation for learning the skills of health assessment.

ASSIGNMENT

CD-ROM content: Chapter 1
Companion website: www.prenhall.com/damico, Chapter 1

VOCABULARY EXERCISE

After completing the reading assignment, you should be able to define the **key terms** listed below. Refer back to the page number from the main text for help.

Charting by exception, 7
Client record, 5
Constant data, 5
Critical thinking, 13–14
Flow sheets, 7
Focus documentation, 7
Focused interview, 4
Formal teaching, 18
Health assessment, 4
Healthy People 2010, 2
HIPAA, 5

Holism, 10
Internal environmental factors, 10
Informal teaching, 18
Interview, 4
Narrative notes, 6
Nursing process, 11
Objective data, 5
Problem-oriented charting, 7
Subjective data, 4
Variable data, 5

STUDY FOCUS

1. Which of the definitions of health presented in Chapter 1 of the text best fits your personal definition of health? Why is it important for the nurse to have a personal definition of health?

2. Greater emphasis is being placed on health promotion today than ever before. What do you see as the benefits of this shift from disease-oriented healthcare? Do you perceive any dangers to the client?

3. In taking a health history, what is the difference between an interview and a focused interview?

4. With whom may the nurse share information from the health record of a client? Does being a healthcare provider entitle one to review any health record at will? What, if any, protection does the client have for information contained in the health record?

5. What is the basic difference in information contained in the health history as compared to the physical assessment record?

6. List one advantage and one disadvantage of the following formats for recording of client data: problem oriented, focus notes, narrative notes, charting by exception, flow sheets, check sheets.

7. How does the nursing process differ from the scientific method? In the evaluation phase, what exactly is evaluated?

8. As the nurse prepares to teach a client about his or her care or condition, what are the elements of a sound teaching plan?

9. Which of the roles of the professional nurse drew you to want to become a nurse? Would more than one of the roles be implemented concurrently by one nurse at any given time?

REVIEW QUESTIONS

1. When client data indicates a special risk of cardiovascular disease and the nurse prepares to teach the client about diet, exercise, and smoking avoidance, the nurse is focusing on

   a. illness and symptoms.
   b. health maintenance.
   c. specific prevention.
   d. general population recommendations.

2. *Healthy People 2010* proposes objectives to improve health specific to identified needs in the U.S. population. Leading health indicators include (Check all that apply.)
   a. cardiovascular disease.
   b. overweight and obesity.
   c. cancer.
   d. sexually transmitted diseases.

3. A client complains of a "cough that is driving me crazy." The nurse must now implement
   a. referral to a physician.
   b. teaching about cough hygiene to prevent spread of microorganisms.
   c. a focused interview.
   d. documentation of a productive cough.

4. Quotation marks are employed in the client record to indicate
   a. casual language.
   b. verbal orders from a physician.
   c. client history in client's own words.
   d. information that has not been confirmed.

5. Which of the following is the difference between charting by exception and focus documentation?
   a. Strengths and problems are included in focus charting.
   b. Both focus on selected problems.
   c. Charting by exception allows repetition of data.
   d. Background data is eliminated in focus charting.

Identify each piece of data as subjective (S) or objective (O).

6. headache occurring in the occipital area _____

7. cough _____

8. blood pressure of 124/82 _____

9. father dying of cardiac arrest at age 46 _____

10. eating a good diet _____

11. appendectomy in 2001 _____

12. Communication occurs through
    a. verbal interaction.
    b. nonverbal interactions.
    c. client records.
    d. professional literature.
    e. all of the above.

13. Mr. Jones is admitted to the hospital for complaints of fatigue and irritability. His lab reports indicate that he is anemic. In the nursing process, this data is part of the step of
    a. assessment.
    b. diagnosis.
    c. planning.
    d. intervention.
    e. evaluation.

14. In planning for Mr. Jones's care, the nurse designs a teaching plan for a healthy diet. The first step in this teaching plan should be
    a. identification of iron-rich foods.
    b. discovering Mr. Jones's food preferences.
    c. obtaining written information for Mr. Jones to take home.
    d. identification of Mr. Jones's knowledge of healthy diet.

15. In assessing a 35-year-old newly admitted mother of three school-age children, the nurse finds the client more anxious about the care of her children than of herself. This is an example of
    a. denial of health threat.
    b. developmentally appropriate response.
    c. failure of the nurse to alleviate client anxiety.
    d. role distortion.

CASE STUDIES

1. Ms. Foster is the school nurse for Strong Elementary School, grades one through six. Part of her job is to develop and review health records for the school's 800 students. In doing this, Ms. Foster has found that the average weight for students is in the 85th percentile and that the physical education program has been eliminated in a cost-cutting move. The school is located in an urban environment, in a neighborhood bordering an industrial area.

   • What are the identified problems of this population?

   • Of what relevance is the document *Healthy People 2010*?

   • How might Ms. Foster use this document in her work?

   • With assessment factors identified, what is the next step in the nursing process?

   • What might be some reasonable short-term goals for Strong students?

   • What short-term goals would be desirable?

- Select one of the identified problems and suggest a plan of care based on short- and long-term goals.

- In her work as a school nurse, what roles would Ms. Foster be implementing?

2. Johnny Jones is a new fourth-grade student at Strong Elementary, where Ms. Foster is the school nurse. In performing an initial health exam, Ms. Foster discovers that Johnny's weight is in the 90th percentile. In the health interview, Johnny reveals that all his family members are "big people." He feels OK, he tells the nurse, but he does report being teased for being so big and he does not like this at all. He states that he is not good at any sport but thinks he will be good at football because "being big is an advantage in football." Johnny states that his mother cooks for him and his family and that she is a really good cook.

   - In the health history interview, what questions would need to be asked of Johnny?

   - What questions would be asked in the focused interview?

   - What risks exist for Johnny related to his obese status?

   - What positive factors exist for Johnny?

   - What would the nurse need to know before planning to change Johnny's eating habits?

   - What factors from the health assessment should be reflected on Johnny's health record?

   - Which of the formats for documentation presented in the textbook would be a good choice for this case? Give a rationale for your choice.

CLINICAL ACTIVITIES

In lab, work alone on the case studies offered here. When you and your lab partner have both finished, take turns presenting your findings to each other. Combine insights and interventions so that you have the best of both efforts in one study.

Wellness and Health Promotion 2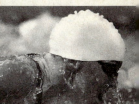

OVERVIEW

This chapter prepares you to address wellness and health promotion, by defining these terms and providing resources for your introduction and understanding. At all levels of client health, the nurse strives to promote health and protect wellness. Such nursing interventions must be grounded in accepted theories and guided by tested principles.

ASSIGNMENT

CD-ROM content: Chapter 2
Companion website: www.prenhall.com/damico, Chapter 2

VOCABULARY EXERCISE

After completing the reading assignment, you should be able to define the **key terms** listed below. Refer back to the page number from the main text for help.

Aerobic exercise, 32
Anaerobic exercise, 32
Biology, 29
Health promotion, 25
Healthy People 2010, 28
Leading health indicators, 29

Physical environment, 29
Primary prevention, 23
Secondary prevention, 24
Social environment, 29
Tertiary prevention, 24

STUDY FOCUS

1. What is meant by the wellness-illness continuum? Can the patient move along the continuum in more than one direction? How does nursing practice relate to this concept?

2. What is your definition of wellness? What are your personal goals for wellness? What are some ways your personal view of wellness could affect your client care, positively or negatively?

3. List the 10 areas of concern identified in *Healthy People 2010.* Are you surprised by these selections for focus? Which of the factors seems to be of greatest concern in your community?

4. What are some reasons adults have for failing to engage in aerobic activity? Do children generally meet recommendations for aerobic activity? What are some reasons that children may fail to meet activity recommendations?

5. During assessment of a client, in what phase of data gathering would the nurse likely identify client failure to meet recommendations for a healthy lifestyle?

6. Which of the 10 areas of concern seem directly related to others? For example, substance abuse seems directly related to injury and violence because most substances abused increase impulsive behavior and decrease coordination. Are there others so related?

REVIEW QUESTIONS

1. Which model employs the concept of levels of actions that promote health, identify and treat disease, and restore health, following disease or trauma?
   a. Dunn
   b. Leavell and Clark
   c. Travis

2. An adolescent is treated in the emergency room for injuries sustained in a skateboard accident. He refuses to wear a helmet, saying, "I'm too good to get seriously hurt." In the health belief model, which perception of the client's is predictive of the likeliness of his taking corrective action?
   a. seriousness of effects of outcome
   b. activity-related effect
   c. cost of reducing risk (helmet)
   d. effectiveness of intervention

3. As the nurse is beginning to encourage the client to engage in some form of exercise, the client interrupts and says, "I tried to run some years ago and I hated it!" According to the health promotion model, this statement relates to
   a. self-efficacy.
   b. perceived benefits of action.
   c. perceptions of available options.
   d. activity-related affect.

4. The document and initiative *Healthy People 2010* is designed to
   a. provide the U.S. Public Health Service with a program target.
   b. identify health problems for medical response planning.
   c. improve the health of communities through individuals.
   d. provide the insurance industry with risk data.

5. Access to healthcare is a health indicator that is related to
   a. adequate numbers of providers.
   b. availability of health insurance.
   c. transportation.
   d. financial resources.
   e. all of the above.

6. *Healthy People 2010* recommendations for school-age children regarding physical activity are
   a. 30 minutes on 5 or more days of the week.
   b. moderate physical activity for 30 minutes 5 days a week and vigorous activity 3 days a week.
   c. vigorous activity 3 or more days per week.
   d. 30 to 60 minutes of activity seven days a week.

7. Asking a client about tobacco use is important because (circle all that apply)
   a. there are many forms of tobacco use, all damaging to health.
   b. many tobacco users would like to quit.
   c. tobacco use can impact medication pharmacokinetics.
   d. it may open discussion of other substance abuse.

8. In order to assist the client with responsible sexual behavior, the nurse would need to know which three basic facts about the client?
   1.
   2.
   3.

9. Mental health problems are concerns of *Healthy People 2010*. Which focused history questions would give the nurse insight about possible depression symptoms for a client?

10. Extreme sports has become a popular phenomenon in the United States. What questions about sport activities could identify risks from such activities?
    1.
    2.
    3.

11. "Who hits who in your family?" is a question suggested for assessment of family violence. This question could (circle all that apply)
    a. communicate to the client that it's OK to discuss physical abuse.
    b. reveal a case of abuse that might be overlooked.
    c. allow the client to confide his or her own abusive tendencies.
    d. offend the client.

Identify the health risk from the *Healthy People 2010* indicators.

12. smoking _____
13. gang activity _____
14. junk food _____
15. non-English-speaking _____
16. sedentary lifestyle _____
17. traffic congestion _____

18. What established tools can be used by the nurse to assess health risks and lifestyle?

19. What tools are available for the client to use in self-assessment? Indicate where these may be found.

20. How many injections are given to the normal 12-month-old infant at the twelve-months well-child visit? How many vaccines does this represent?

CASE STUDIES

1. Nancy is a student nurse who comes to the university health clinic seeking help with her weight gain. Since starting college, she has gained 14 pounds and wants to correct this situation before it becomes an entrenched problem. Nancy is asked to fill out a lifestyle inventory, which reveals the following: she has class 15 hours per week with an additional 12 hours of labs and clinical activities, she commutes 2 hours daily, she studies an average of 20 hours per week and has household duties of 20 hours a week (cleaning, cooking, shopping, laundry, grooming), and she sleeps on average 6 to 7 hours nightly. She smoked a little in high school and not at all her first 2 years in college, but she resumed smoking hoping it would help with the weight gain. She has four cups of coffee and one or two colas daily. The campus is inner city, and she is reluctant to walk many places for safety reasons.

   Using *Healthy People 2010* as a guide, answer the following questions:

   - What are Nancy's real health risks?
   - What are Nancy's potential health risks?
   - How should Nancy's health risks be prioritized for intervention?
   - What would be one reasonable short-term (6 weeks) goal for each of Nancy's health risks?

2. Mrs. Gonzolez has type 2 diabetes in fairly good control. As the nurse compliments her on her blood sugar findings, Mrs. Gonzolez replies, "Yes. I restrict my eating to whatever it takes to keep the blood sugar in line. If it rises during the day I just stop eating." When asked about exercise, Mrs. Gonzolez says she avoids this because it

causes changes in her blood sugar and that she does not know how to adjust for these changes in her eating. She admits to being very frightened about her disease and says that she is often tearful when thinking about the future.

- What additional information would you like to have based on this interview?

Using *Healthy People 2010* as a guide, answer the following questions:

- What are Mrs. Gonzolez's real health risks?

- What are some potential health risks?

- What type of nursing intervention should play a major role in Mrs. Gonzolez's care?

- What levels of prevention are applicable to Mrs. Gonzolez's case?

CLINICAL ACTIVITIES

Take a history from your lab partner or a willing friend. When doing history exercises, it's OK to role-play rather than having to reveal personal facts that may be better kept private. If you do role-play, however, try to stay "in character." This means that you do not shift from your adopted role back to your own life facts. For example, if you role-play a teenager with a sedentary lifestyle, don't mention that you have leg cramps after running more than 3 miles!

▸ Ask the basic health history questions and look for the indicators mentioned in *Healthy People 2010*.
▸ List any such indicators and brainstorm with your client about why these factors exist and what changes might be made.
▸ Document the indicators and list interventions that your client agrees to adopt.

Reverse roles and be a client for your partner.

WELLNESS AND HEALTH PROMOTION ASSESSMENT

Using the sample documentation forms at the end of the chapter as a guideline:

- Perform a wellness and health promotion assessment.
- Ensure your client's comfort and privacy as you ask these questions.
- Reassure the client as to the confidentiality of his or her responses and the usefulness of the information being gathered.

NURSING DIAGNOSIS

Look through the nursing diagnoses in **Appendix A of your text**. How many of the nursing diagnoses relate directly to health and health promotion, rather than disease? Think about the meaning of this in terms of the domain of nursing.

Sample Documentation Form

Assessment of Wellness and Health Promotion

Name: _____ Date: _____

Age: _____ Gender: _____

History
Client's own statement of wellness: _____
_____

Primary Prevention
   Specific prevention (immunizations, safety precautions for occupation, recreation, transportation):
   _____
   _____

   Health promotion (efforts at healthy diet, exercise, stress reduction, socialization, sleep, hygiene):
   _____
   _____

   Prepathologic signs (if any): _____
   _____

Secondary Prevention
   Screening (see Chapter 3 in your text for age-specific recommendations for screening): _____
   _____

   Identified illness: _____
   _____

Treatment in progress or treatment needed: _____
_____

Tertiary Prevention (Rehabilitation Needs): _____
_____

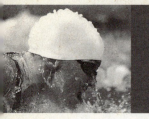

3 Health Assessment Across the Life Span

OVERVIEW

This chapter will help you review with the many facets of growth and development and their application to expert health assessment and excellent nursing care. Just as with all aspects of assessment, there are norms of growth and development, and clients are assessed according to the norms of their expected developmental level. In order to do assessments of each client's growth and development, the nurse must have knowledge of biological, psychosocial, intellectual, and spiritual norms.

ASSIGNMENT

CD-ROM content: Chapter 3
Companion website: www.prenhall.com/damico, Chapter 3, especially Toolbox

VOCABULARY EXERCISE

After completing the reading assignment, you should be able to define the **key terms** listed below. Refer back to the page number from the main text for help.

Adolescence, 58
Cephalocaudal, 47
Cognitive theory, 48
Development, 47
Growth, 47
Infant, 49
Middle adulthood, 61

Older adult, 63
Preschooler, 54
Psychoanalytic theory, 48
Psychosocial theory, 49
School age, 56
Toddler, 52
Young adult, 61

STUDY FOCUS

1. In assessing an 18-month-old child, his ability to pick up a raisin placed in front of him is important. What aspect of development does this ability represent? Which developmental theorist presented in your textbook speaks to this skill directly?

2. Safety issues in the first years of life include concern about any object small enough to be placed in an infant's or a toddler's mouth. The nurse will want to make teaching about choking hazards an important part of teaching to new parents. Which theorist explains this stage of infant behavior most directly?

3. All theories of psychosocial development acknowledge the importance of the extent to which a child's needs are met. List three behaviors of a mother and child that can be observed by the nurse during a well-child visit that could be used to assess the degree of attachment of mother and child. What health concerns might arise should attachment be impaired?

4. What are some possible nursing diagnoses for a child of 3 years who is unable to pedal a tricycle or climb stairs using alternate feet? What questions would you ask the parent or caregiver of this child? What nursing interventions could be suggested?

5. In adolescence, children want to rely on their own reasoning and to problem solve for themselves. What behaviors might give evidence of such development? What are some hazards of this stage based on this desirable progress? What teaching might the nurse do with parents of children in this stage?

6. Young adults are expected to be in their prime of health and beginning competence. What are some activities of daily living that may become unhealthy during this stage? Why would this be the case? What nursing interventions related to diet and exercise become important now?

7. This generation of middle adults has additional stressors in caring for children longer and taking on responsibilities of aging parents at the same time. What are some self-care behaviors that might suffer at this stage? In the role of referral agent, what are some suggestions the nurse might make to the client experiencing such burdens? What mental health issues might be of concern for these clients?

8. In assessment of frail older adults, which non-disease-state physical factors become of concern? Which emotional health factors have potential for physical illness?

REVIEW QUESTIONS

1. Development proceeds from _____ to _____. In turn, differentiated development begins with a generalized response and proceeds to a _____.

2. Children age 7 to 11 love to play board games, such as Monopoly. They generally learn the rules well and become meticulous about enforcing rules of any game. This is because they are in
   a. an ego dominant stage.
   b. a preoperational stage.
   c. a concrete operational stage.
   d. a superego stage of intense conscience.

3. Cries of "Daddy will dress me" and "I want to go with Daddy" can represent
   a. a phallic stage.
   b. an initiative stage.
   c. a preoperational egocentric stage.
   d. a failure to bond with mother.

4. Baby Smith is boisterous, social, and energetic. Her mother is quiet and somewhat shy. Mom tells you that baby is "a character and more fun than I ever could have imagined." Mom and baby have
   a. goodness of fit.
   b. hurdles to overcome.
   c. a potential for bonding problems.
   d. a potential for abuse.

5. A child who can skip on one foot, catch a ball with two hands, cut a straight line with scissors, and try to put puzzles together is _____ years of age.

6. The most rapid growth during the school years occurs in the
   a. cardiovascular system.
   b. neurologic system.
   c. skeletal system.
   d. reproductive system.

7. Many adolescents dress in a manner and style that is unlike their adult social group. This is usually evidence of
   a. searching for identity.
   b. increasing independence from parents.
   c. forming a value system.
   d. developing a sexual identity.

8. High-risk sexual behavior is life threatening in
   a. adolescence.
   b. young adulthood.
   c. middle adulthood.
   d. middle-aged adults.
   e. all of the above.

9. Loneliness in older adults due to loss of spouse or friends can manifest as
   a. depression.
   b. poor nutrition.
   c. regression.
   d. confusion.
   e. a and b.

10. Protection of cognitive function in older adults is significantly affected by _____.

CASE STUDIES

1. Alexandra, 4 years of age, is going to get a new sister at her house. Her mother is wondering how and when to tell Alexandra about the new baby and what aspects of the baby's care Alexandra might be able to do.

   - According to Erikson, how capable is Alexandra of focusing on a baby?

   - How likely is she to understand the concept of the baby coming in 8 months? On what do you base your opinion?

   - Is it reasonable to think that Alexandra can provide some care for the new baby? What aspects of the new baby's care could Alexandra do? On what do you base your opinion?

   - According to psychoanalytic theory, what concerns might the parents have regarding Alexandra and the new baby?

2. Mr. Jasper is a 72-year-old widower who lives alone. His health is reasonable for his age, but he does have frequent headaches and type 2 diabetes. He is in the hospital today for observation following a fall in his kitchen. No fractures

are found, and he will most likely be going home today or tomorrow. He has asked some of the same questions over and over, and you are beginning to wonder about confusion.

- What are some screening procedures that you can do to clarify Mr. Jasper's status? List all that seem reasonable.

- What questions do you have about Mr. Jasper's medical conditions?

- What focused history would you see as necessary?

- What health promotion concerns do you have for Mr. Jasper?

CLINICAL ACTIVITIES

In your lab group there are likely to be persons of different developmental levels, along with persons who have grandparents or elderly neighbors, and who are parents of children of various ages. Break into small groups and refer to the boxes in Chapter 3 of your text. These boxes give great detail on interventions for each age group.

Taking each box in turn, discuss the interventions as to what you have observed of your friends and children.

- Do the interventions seem appropriate for the persons your group has knowledge of? For example, one population intervention for clients age 65 and older is to assess for risk of falls. Do you see this in your experience?

DEVELOPMENTAL ASSESSMENT

Using the sample documentation form at the end of the chapter as a guideline, perform a developmental assessment.

- Ensure your client's comfort and privacy as you ask these very personal questions.
- Reassure the client as to the confidentiality of his or her responses and the usefulness of the information being gathered.
- If your client is too young, too ill, or too compromised to answer these questions, seek a significant other or a caretaker to provide needed information.

NURSING DIAGNOSIS

Look through the nursing diagnoses in **Appendix A of your text**. How many of the nursing diagnoses relate directly to growth and development? This emphasis reflects the importance of considering growth and development norms while caring for clients of all ages.

Sample Documentation Form

Health Assessment Across the Life Span

Name: _____ Date: _____

Age: _____ Gender: _____

Developmental Assessment

Select models appropriate for the chronological age of the client and assess the following:

Physical Growth

Height: _____ Weight: _____ Additional anthropometric measurements relative to age:

_____

_____

Motor functioning (coordination, balance, gait): _____

_____

Language ability: _____

Cognitive functioning (level of education): _____

_____

Psychosocial functioning (interpersonal relationships, work, school): _____

_____

Sleep/rest/stress-reduction patterns: _____

_____

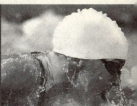

4

OVERVIEW

Chapter 4 presents information about the concept of culture and its impact on health and healthcare. It also offers a wealth of information about specific cultures demonstrating diverse cultural phenomena. This knowledge is critical to the nursing assessment of clients and impacts the ability of the nurse to relate to the client. Knowledge of a client's culture assists the nurse in establishing a workable relationship with the client and in planning and carrying out care that is acceptable to the client.

ASSIGNMENT

CD-ROM content: Chapter 4
Companion website: www.prenhall.com/damico, Chapter 4, especially Toolbox

VOCABULARY EXERCISE

After completing the reading assignment, you should be able to define the **key terms** listed below. Refer back to the page number from the main text for help.

Assimilation, 72
Cultural competence, 70
Culture, 70
Diversity, 72
Ethnicity, 72

Ethnocentrism, 72
Nonverbal communication, 76
Race, 72
Subculture, 71
Verbal communication, 76

STUDY FOCUS

1. The commitment of the nurse to promote and support the attitudes, behaviors, knowledge, and skills necessary for staff to work respectfully and effectively with clients and each other in a culturally diverse work setting is a laudable one. Is it entirely up to the personal taste of the nurse to make this commitment? Why is the word *staff* included in this commitment?

2. What is the difference between ethnicity and race? Do both of these concepts have cultural elements?

3. Other than actual language, what are some aspects of communication that vary significantly according to culture?

4. What are the main family patterns that are seen in the assessment of cultures? How does the position of power vary among Arab, Appalachian, and African Americans?

5. Silence is a form of nonverbal communication that ranges from supportive to hostile and from respectful to disrespectful. How many ways can silence be used to communicate?

6. How can cultural orientation to time affect responses to healthcare? How can it affect treatment itself?

REVIEW QUESTIONS

1. The capacity of nurses or health services delivery systems to effectively understand and plan for the needs of a culturally diverse client or group is referred to as
   a. cultural assimilation.
   b. ethnocentrism.
   c. cultural competence.
   d. ethnic diversity.

2. Give some examples of material culture.

3. A term for a group of people who share a common culture and who belong to a specific group that holds similar values is
   a. race.
   b. ethnicity.
   c. subculture.
   d. sect.
   e. geopolitical group.

4. Assimilation is a culturally based choice required of nurses in order to give culturally competent care.
   a. true
   b. false

5. Cultural phenomena that are part of the Chinese American culture include which of the following?
   a. Time references are present oriented.
   b. Diet is high in fat and starch.
   c. Health is associated with moderate obesity.
   d. The power base is matrilineal.
   e. Traditional medicine is the initial and preferred choice.

6. Cultures that believe illness is God's will may present problems of
   a. noncompliance with treatment.
   b. fatalism.
   c. lack of motivation for health promotion.
   d. guilt associated with condition.
   e. all of the above.

7. Folk healing has no quality control standards and thus
   a. is a dangerous practice.
   b. must be evaluated in practice.
   c. is probably harmless.
   d. must be forbidden in scientific medical treatment.

8. List concerns the nurse must have when caring for clients who do not share the nurse's language.

CASE STUDIES

1. Few nurses would knowingly exhibit ethnocentrism. However, many of our intensely held beliefs are, indeed, cultural values. For example, the nurse in contemporary American society may balk at the idea that a female client believes she must seek permission from her mother-in-law to receive treatment for cancer. What are some ways the nurse could reconcile this disparity of beliefs and give culturally competent care?

2. Referring to Table 4.1 in your text, discuss the differences in approach to a Jewish American client as compared to a Filipino American with regard to planning and offering health promotion interventions.

CLINICAL ACTIVITIES

If possible, invite members of two or three local cultures to speak to your lab group about their culture, specifically their health beliefs.

▶ Be sure to prepare for this seminar by reading material in Chapter 4 of your textbook.

▶ Give each speaker a list of cultural phenomena presented in your book (communication, temporal relations, dietary habits, family patterns, health beliefs, health practices) so that there are points of comparison for your discussions.

CULTURAL ASSESSMENT

Using the sample documentation form at the end of this chapter as a guideline, perform a cultural assessment.

▶ Ensure your client's comfort and privacy as you ask these very personal questions.
▶ Reassure the client as to the confidentiality of his or her responses and the usefulness of the information being gathered.
▶ Be very careful with documentation you make during this exercise. If this is a real client, your documentation will become part of the protected chart. If this is a volunteer, be sure to dispose of the record in a way that will not allow it to be seen by anyone other than yourself, your partner, or your nursing teacher.

NURSING DIAGNOSIS

Look through the nursing diagnoses in **Appendix A of your text**. How many of the nursing diagnoses relate directly to cultural situations? Look again and see if some of the diagnoses would be affected by cultural differences. For example, situations dealing with communication, nutrition, and relationships could be greatly affected by cultural factors if the client and the nurse come from different cultures. Parenting, coping, and even pain management could be affected by cultural differences. Discuss various possibilities with your lab partner and classmates. Sharing cultural perspectives with others can help to enlarge your appreciation of diverse perspectives.

Sample Documentation Form

Cultural Assessment

Name: _____ Date: _____

Age: _____ Gender: _____

Document observations and statements by the client.

Language(s)   Primary: _____ Other: _____

Embraced culture (culture stated by client): _____

Subculture (can be ethnic, professional, religious, etc.): _____
_____

Family patterns (authority figures, roles of client): _____
_____

Health beliefs (causes of illness/wellness): _____
_____

Health practices (use of healers, medications, alternative treatments): _____
_____

Dietary habits (in health and illness): _____
_____

Communication patterns (verbal and nonverbal, touch, allowed topics): _____
_____
_____

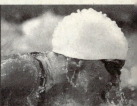

OVERVIEW

This chapter provides you with tools and an approach to assess the psychosocial functioning of clients. The psychosocial domain is a huge part of life and impacts all other aspects of functioning. This assessment requires great tact and perceptiveness on the part of the nurse but yields information crucial to the effectiveness of nursing interventions.

ASSIGNMENT

CD-ROM content: Chapter 5
Companion website: www.prenhall.com/damico, Chapter 5

VOCABULARY EXERCISE

After completing the reading assignment, you should be able to define the **key terms** listed below. Refer back to the page number from the main text for help.

Interdependent relationships, 84
Psychosocial functioning, 81
Psychosocial health, 81

Role development, 84
Self-concept, 83
Stress, 82

STUDY FOCUS

1. What are the components of psychosocial health? How does this differ from psychosocial functioning?

2. What genetic influences affect psychosocial health? Because an influence is genetic, is there any intervention that can change the outcome?

3. Physical fitness clearly impacts physical health. Does it have an identifiable effect on psychosocial health? What are some of the common effects lack of physical fitness can have on psychosocial health?

4. Economic status can prevent persons from obtaining healthcare when needed. What are some basic needs that can be directly affected by economic status? What health promotion factors can be affected by economic status?

5. List three family behaviors that directly influence psychosocial functioning. In what way can the professional nurse hope to make an impact on family functioning?

6. What are some signs of a positive self-concept in a client? What are some signs of a negative self-concept?

7. Of what value is a client's positive self-concept to the nurse who wishes to offer physical care? How can the client's self-concept affect compliance to a treatment regimen?

8. The ability to form relationships is addressed by developmental theorists. Review this section in Chapter 3 and identify which of the developmental theorists uses this ability as a landmark of development.

9. Define stress. Is there more than one kind of stress?

10. Identify a tool for spiritual assessment presented in Chapter 5 of your text.

REVIEW QUESTIONS

1. Where can information for psychosocial assessment be obtained?
   a. medical record
   b. client interview
   c. family interview/report
   d. physical assessment
   e. all of the above

2. Psychosocial well-being is established in early development and remains relatively unchanged throughout life.
   a. true
   b. false

3. List focused interview questions the nurse could ask if suspicious that a client suffers from low self-esteem.

4. List at least four red flags for the possibility of psychosocial dysfunction.

5. How might diabetes mellitus affect psychosocial functioning? Give a brief discussion.

6. Conflict between societal norms and personal choices can lead to psychosocial dysfunction. Identify two such choices that could lead to psychosocial stress in contemporary society.

7. Which of the following should alert the nurse to psychosocial dysfunction? Circle all that apply.
   a. extreme sports
   b. lack of time for recreation
   c. economic change for the better
   d. competitive gaming
   e. gambling

8. Mental health dysfunctions may come to light during the focused interview. List three aspects of assessment that indicate sound brain functioning.

9. In order to fairly test a client's orientation to judgment and attention span, it is essential to have knowledge of the client's (circle all that apply)
   a. culture.
   b. educational level.
   c. language.
   d. family orientation.

10. Abnormal speech patterns may indicate
    a. anxiety.
    b. neurologic impairment.
    c. lying.
    d. depression.
    e. all of the above.

CASE STUDIES

1. Consider what impact even minor physical illness may have on psychosocial health. For example, a 3-day fever might have what impact on a busy student nurse?

   • List the actual impact such an illness may make to the student's schedule.

   • Now list at least three psychosocial reactions to physical illness.

   • What negative outcomes could be foreseen?

   • What nursing interventions could be suggested?

   • What outcomes would be desirable?

2. Thomas is a 13-year-old who has been homeless with his mother for the last 2 years. He is enrolled in the seventh grade at a middle school and sleeps in a family shelter. He must be out of the shelter at 7 a.m. and may not return until 6 p.m. His school opens at 8:30 a.m., but most school buses do not arrive until 9 a.m. and classes start at 9:15 a.m.

   • Given Thomas's developmental level, what are likely threats to his self-esteem?

   • What physical changes is he likely facing? What are his resources for dealing with these changes?

- What concerns do you have for his physical health? His health promotion activities?

- What concerns do you have for his psychosocial health and functioning?

ASSESSMENT OF PSYCHOSOCIAL FUNCTIONING

Using the sample documentation form at the end of the chapter as a guideline, perform a psychosocial assessment.

▸ Ensure your client's comfort and privacy as you ask very personal questions.
▸ Reassure the client as to the confidentiality of his or her responses and the usefulness of the information being gathered. If this is a real client, your documentation will become part of the protected chart. If this is a volunteer, be sure to dispose of the record in a way that will not allow it to be seen by anyone other than yourself, your partner, or your nursing teacher.

NURSING DIAGNOSIS

Look through the nursing diagnoses in **Appendix A of your text**. How many of the nursing diagnoses relate directly to psychosocial dynamics? How often could psychosocial diagnoses be combined with physiological diagnoses? What does this tell you about the focus of nursing care?

Sample Documentation Form

Psychosocial Assessment

Name: _____ Date: _____

Age: _____ Gender: _____

Developmental level: _____

Family status: _____

Culture: _____

Economic status: _____

Assessment of self-concept: _____

Role: _____ Role development: _____

Relationships: _____

Spiritual and belief patterns: _____

Stress and coping: _____

Health-promotion beliefs: _____

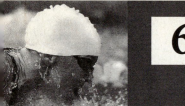

6   Techniques and Equipment

OVERVIEW

This chapter will introduce you to the four techniques used in physical assessment, and the traditional equipment and protocols that enhance those techniques. Physical examination encompasses structure and function and proceeds from the general to the specific, moving from the outside to the inside of the subject. Bilateral symmetry of the body and any of its structures is another crucial assessment.

Examination always begins with **inspection,** which includes not only sight, but smell and listening. For example, the nurse looks at the client and notices that there is an odor about the breath and that the client's voice is hoarse. In all systems but abdominal, **palpation** is the next logical step. Palpation includes feeling for the presence or absence of a structure, determining its form, as well as sensing the temperature, softness or firmness, and texture in question.

Having carefully looked at and touched the subject, the technique of **percussion** is employed to discover the density of tissue being examined. Tapping on the body and listening to the sound generated can help reveal underlying tissue to be air or fluid filled, semisolid muscle, or solid bone. Finally, **auscultation** is used to amplify the sound the body is making on its own. Today, this can be accomplished with a stethoscope or a Doppler.

All of the diagnostic equipment used in examination, from the simplest to the most technologically advanced, simply enhances the basic techniques of examination. For example, ophthalmoscopes and otoscopes improve the ability to inspect areas not readily available to the unassisted eye. Dopplers and electronic stethoscopes improve the ability to hear the sounds the body is making. Thermometers are more accurate in measuring temperature than the nurse's hand might be in assessing fever. It is therefore important to learn the use and limitations of the common tools of assessment so that the most accurate assessments can be made.

ASSIGNMENT

CD-ROM content: Chapter 6
Companion website: www.prenhall.com/damico, Chapter 6

VOCABULARY EXERCISE

After completing the reading assignment, you should be able to define the **key terms** listed below. Refer back to the page number from the main text for help.

Auscultation, 100
Cues, 105
Database, 96
Dullness, 100
Flatness, 100
Fremitus, 97
Hyperresonance, 100

Inspection, 96
Palpation, 100
Percussion, 98
Pleximeter, 99
Plexor, 99
Resonance, 100
Tympany, 100

STUDY FOCUS

1. Describe the techniques of physical assessment and give one example of an expected or unexpected finding discovered by use of each technique.
   Inspection:
   Palpation:
   Percussion:
   Auscultation:

2. In assessment of an abdominal complaint, which type(s) of palpation would you expect to use? Why?

3. Why would you not want to percuss over bone?

4. What are the principal concerns in the use of the stethoscope? Consider use **and** care. When would you especially want the use of a Doppler stethoscope?

5. Why would a grid setting be useful on an ophthalmoscope setting?

6. Are nurses detectives? **What** relevance are cues?

7. How would you conduct a physical assessment of a Saudi woman who believes she should not disrobe for a stranger?

8. What specific information is given by the Centers for Disease Control (link at Companion Website for your text) for protection of the nurse during assessment and treatment?

REVIEW QUESTIONS

1. Inspection may be performed using (circle all that apply)
   a. simple observation.
   b. instrumentation such as x-ray.
   c. a stethoscope.
   d. an ophthalmoscope.
   e. weight scales.
   f. a goniometer.

2. Fremitus is
   a. an expected finding on the abdomen.
   b. detected on palpation.
   c. a pulsation on the chest wall.
   d. a technique of precise measurement.

3. Differentiate between light and moderate palpation and indicate when each would be used.

4. The purpose of indirect percussion is to
   a. produce a clearer sound.
   b. protect underlying tissue.

5. A percussion sound associated with an empty stomach is
   a. tympany.
   b. resonance.
   c. hyperresonance.
   d. dullness.
   e. flatness.

6. The length of the tubing on a stethoscope affects
   a. quality of sound.
   b. type of sound.
   c. duration of sound.

7. List the descriptors used for auscultated sounds.

   _____

   _____

   _____

   _____

8. The bell of the stethoscopic head is best at detecting _____ pitched sounds.

9. Drapes are used for the client during examination to provide for _____ and for _____ .

CLINICAL ACTIVITIES

1. Familiarize yourself with the techniques of examination.

   In the privacy of your room, practice the techniques of examination on yourself. Choose an aspect of your body to **inspect,** for example, your chest.

Inspection

▶ Observe its shape and the contour of the ribs, sternum, and clavicle.
▶ Observe its movement as you breathe in and out.
▶ Inspect the color of the skin.

Palpation

▶ Palpate the skin lightly for texture and temperature.
▶ Palpate muscles for presence, symmetry, and lesions.
▶ Palpate ribs, sternum, and clavicle for tenderness and lesions.

Percussion

▶ Use indirect percussion. Take care to percuss over soft tissue, not bone.
▶ Percuss over your chest and listen to the sounds. Are the sounds the same everywhere?

Auscultation

▶ Use the diaphragm of your stethoscope.
▶ Listen to your breath as you breathe naturally in and then out.
▶ Do inspiration and expiration sound the same?
▶ Listen close to your sternum, then listen down toward the bases of the lungs. Do you note a difference?

2. Spend time with your lab partner examining the various pieces of equipment presented in Chapter 6 of your text.

▶ Try your stethoscope on for comfort. Most come with a small selection of earpieces. Try each, until the earpieces are comfortable for you.
▶ Listen to your own heartbeat with the bell of the stethoscope. Now listen with the diaphragm. What difference, if any, do you detect?
▶ Take the ophthalmoscope and turn it on so that it shines on your upturned hand. Rotate the aperture control so that you can see each of the options for viewing. Note the grid, the colors, and the size of the options.
▶ Open the goniometer and lay it along your arm, from upper arm to lower arm on the inner aspect. Bend your elbow to form an angle. Now bend the goniometer to conform to your elbow angle. Read the goniometer measurement. This is a direct measurement of your joint angle.

Note: See the Fact Sheet that follows this chapter for additional considerations and information on techniques of physical assessment.

Review Appendices B and C in your text for essential information on preventing contamination of equipment of all kinds. This care is of utmost importance to the protection of the client and the nurse in all activities of nursing care.

Assessment Techniques Fact Sheet

Inspection:

- Some have said that 80% of all assessment occurs with observation.
- Observe the client's affect, behavior, hygiene, eye contact, and nonverbal language.
- Some instruments—such as a penlight or goose-neck lamp, otoscope, or ophthalmoscope—may be used to enhance inspection.
- As inspection is done, visualize the underlying anatomical structures.
- Ensure time to collect the observation data before beginning to ask questions or touch the client.
- Document observations, not judgments. For example, "The client has slurred speech and tremor," not "The client appears intoxicated."

Palpation:

Protect the nurse with gloves before touching any area that might have blood and/or body fluids.

- Ensure clean and warm hands before touching the client.
- The finger pads, bases of the fingers, and ulnar surface of the hand all are used during palpation.
- Use the finger pads to determine skin moisture, organ position and characteristics, size and consistency of tissue, pain, and masses.
- The bases of the fingers, as well as the ulnar surface of the hand, are used to feel vibrations.
- Be systematic in the approach. Develop a stepwise palpation routine and use that routine each time the client is assessed.
- During palpation, visualize the underlying anatomical structures.
- Use light, moderate, or deep palpation as appropriate to body area.
- Document location of palpated finding, size and consistency of tissue, and whether tenderness or pain was elicited by palpation.

Percussion: Sounds Made by Striking the Body

Direct Percussion

- The technique involves tapping the body with the fingertips of the dominant hand.

Indirect Percussion

- The technique involves the middle finger of the examiner's nondominant hand being placed firmly on the client's body surface (the pleximeter).
- The middle finger of the dominant hand is used as the striking hand. The examiner's wrist of the dominant hand is held close to the client's skin. The wrist is cocked, and then the plexor rapidly taps or hammers down on the stationary finger on the skin's surface. The result is a subtle but distinctive sound that describes the underlying structure.
- Take care to keep the wrist of the "striking hand" loose and flexible. The tapping motion should be from a flick of the wrist and NOT a hammer motion from the elbow.
- Sounds generated are comparable to direct percussion and may produce a clear sound.
- Indirect percussion is often used over larger body surfaces.

Percussion Tones	Location
Resonant	Lungs
Flat	Bones and muscles
Dull	Solid organs
Tympanic	Stomach and bowels

Blunt percussion is a special and distinct technique designed to cause percussive disturbance to underlying tissue—usually the kidneys—to determine tenderness not discernible on palpation.

Document location percussed and tone heard on percussion.

Auscultation: Sounds Made by the Body

- The acoustic, or Doppler, stethoscope is used for auscultation.
- The acoustic stethoscope should be of professional quality and should have both a bell and a diaphragm.
- The bell is used to detect low-pitched sounds.
- The diaphragm is used to detect high-pitched sounds.
- Whenever auscultating tones, note the sound intensity, pitch, duration, and quality.
- The size of the bell and diaphragm should be appropriate for the size of the client. For example, when working with infants or very young children, a pediatric-size bell and diaphragm is appropriate.
- The tubing of the stethoscope should measure no longer than 30 to 40 cm and at least 4 mm in diameter.
- Its function is to screen out room noise and to direct sound from the end piece to the nurse's ear.
- The earpieces should fit comfortably and snugly in your ear canal. When inserting, be sure to angle them toward your nose so that the sound is more clearly transmitted to your tympanic membranes.

Document location auscultated and findings identified.

General Survey 7

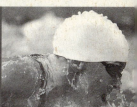

OVERVIEW

This chapter presents the general appraisal, which is an educated first impression of the client. The general appraisal opens the door to more specific assessment techniques but is, itself, a professional appraisal that is the foundation of and guide to further evaluation. No doubt, many times you have approached a friend and had the distinct feeling that your friend is not feeling well or is uncomfortable in some way. The educated general survey expands upon this "feeling" by guiding focus in an organized way and comparing client features to expected standards.

ASSIGNMENT

CD-ROM content: Chapter 7
Companion website: www.prenhall.com/damico, Chapter 7

VOCABULARY EXERCISE

After completing the reading assignment, you should be able to define the **key terms** listed below. Refer back to the page number from the main text for help.

Blood pressure, 116
Functional assessment, 120
General survey, 109
Hyperthermia, 113
Hypothermia, 113
Oxygen saturation, 116
Pain, 119

Pain rating scale, 119
Pulse, 114
Respiratory rate, 116
Sphygmomanometer, 117
Temperature, 113
Vital signs, 113

STUDY FOCUS

1. The general survey is indeed general, but it has four specific focuses. What are they?

2. What factors can artificially alter vital signs? Identify one or two of these factors and indicate in what way they can change each vital sign.
    Temperature:
    Pulse:
    Respiratory rate:
    Blood pressure:

3. What is cardiac output and in what way can it affect blood pressure? Pulse?

4. What age-related factors affect temperature in terms of expected findings?

5. Why would pain be considered a vital sign? How might pain affect respiratory rate?

6. What behaviors might be observed in a newly admitted client that would serve as data for a functional assessment?

REVIEW QUESTIONS

1. The nurse observes an adult client dressed warmly in pants, a jacket, and a long-sleeved shirt on a very hot summer day. This observation (circle all that apply)
   a. is part of the general appraisal.
   b. requires follow-up questions.
   c. relates to mental status.
   d. relates to orientation to place.

2. An uneven, halting gait could relate to what factors?
   _____
   _____
   _____

3. An adolescent being seen for a health appraisal would be expected to relate to a parent in the presence of the nurse by being
   a. dependent on the adult for answers to health questions.
   b. unconcerned about the parent.
   c. uncomfortable during questions relating to sexuality.

4. Any client who repeatedly asks for questions to be repeated, seems confused about topics presented, and gives inappropriate information might be suspected of being
   a. mentally compromised.
   b. hard of hearing.
   c. neurologically impaired.
   d. under the influence of medication/drugs.
   e. any of the above.

5. The Metropolitan height and weight charts are corrected for (circle all that apply)
   a. gender.
   b. age.
   c. skeletal frame.
   d. body mass index.
   e. racial characteristics.

6. There are significant age variations in expected temperature:
   a. Older clients tend to have _____ temperatures compared to younger adults.
   b. Children tend to have _____ temperatures compared to adults.
   c. Adolescents tend to have _____ temperatures compared to adults.

7. List the eight sites for common pulse measurement.

8. The following factors tend to result in **lower** pulse rates (circle all that apply):
   a. younger age
   b. adult female
   c. hemorrhage
   d. client (prolonged) standing
   e. client sitting
   f. fever

9. What six factors should always be documented when a pulse is recorded?

10. On measuring vital signs, if the nurse detects irregularities of pulse or respiratory rate, what should be done?

11. List five factors that can impact the blood pressure of a client.

12. If the blood pressure cuff is too large for the client, likely the measurement of blood pressure will be artificially _____.

13. What is the purpose of a palpated blood pressure?

14. In an auscultated blood pressure assessment, the fifth Korotkoff sound represents _____.

15. In an 18-month-old child, which artery should be used to measure blood pressure?

CASE STUDY

1. Myron, a 70-year-old tennis player, comes to the clinic for a checkup. He takes one antihypertensive medication. He is retired, financially stable, and of normal weight for his height. His gait is confident but somewhat uneven as he steps more rapidly on the left leg than on the right. It is a very warm day and you observe him taking a quick drink from the fountain as he comes into the exam room. You begin by taking his vital signs:

   Blood pressure 160/90

   Temperature 100 oral

   Respiratory rate 22, inaudible, even

   Pulse 92

   Why would his blood pressure be elevated if he is taking an antihypertensive medication?

   What are some possible explanations for his temperature reading? His pulse? His respiratory rate?

   What focused interview questions would you ask?

CLINICAL ACTIVITIES

Make a general survey of your client

- ▶ Note gait, manner, attitude, and body language in an organized way.
- ▶ Be aware of the client's level of alertness and orientation to time, self, and place.
- ▶ Prepare needed equipment for assessing vital signs.
- ▶ Take vital signs on your designated client and record as directed by guidelines.

  In the remaining time in lab, take as many of your lab classmates' vital signs as you can.

- ▶ Record findings on the form provided using first names only to provide privacy.
- ▶ Compare recorded vital signs with each other to assess accuracy.
- ▶ If anyone's vital signs are outside expected limits, be sure to call this to the person's attention as privately as possible. Offer to repeat the vital signs for accuracy.

| | | **PULSE:** | | |
| | | **RATE** | | |
NAME	**TEMPERATURE (ROUTE)**	**RHYTHM**	**RESPIRATORY RATE**	**BLOOD PRESSURE**

Vital Signs Recording Form

GENERAL SURVEY AND ASSESSMENT OF VITAL SIGNS

Using the sample documentation form at the end of this chapter as a guideline, perform a general survey and assess the vital signs of a willing volunteer or, if possible, one of your clinical clients. Be sure to take the brief history indicated before measuring the vital signs. How does the history help you put the vital signs in context?

Note the adjusted blood pressure norms for girls in **Appendix D** and for boys in **Appendix E of your text.**

Also, review care of equipment in **Appendix B of your text** to prevent contamination of equipment and exposure of client or nurse to pathogens.

NURSING DIAGNOSIS

Review appendix A in your text. Which nursing diagnoses relate directly to a client's vital signs?

Sample Documentation Form

General Survey and Vital Signs

Name: _____   Date: _____

Age: _____   Gender: _____

Observations

Physical appearance (height and weight proportion, grooming, hygiene, impression):

_____

_____

_____

Mental status (affect, mood appropriateness, orientation, memory, speech):

_____

_____

_____

Neurologic status (gait, coordination, mobility):

_____

_____

_____

Analysis:

_____

_____

_____

_____

History
Review of history related to vital signs:
Medications:

_____

_____

Smoking: _____

Cardiovascular disease: _____

Respiratory disease: _____

Family history of cardiovascular or respiratory disease: _____

_____

_____

Temperature

_____ _____   Recent fever _____

_____ _____   Illness during past week _____

Pulse

_____ _____   Racing or irregular pulse _____

_____ _____   Cardiovascular disease _____

Respirations

____ ____   Respiratory disease _____

____ ____   Breathing difficulties _____

Blood Pressure

____ ____   History of hypertension _____

____ ____   Headaches _____

____ ____   Weakness _____

____ ____   Dizziness _____

Vital Sign Assessment

Vital Sign	Date/Time	Finding	
Temperature Oral Axillary Rectal Tympanic			

Pulse
Rate
Location
Quality
Rhythm
 	
Respirations
Rate
Rhythm
Quality
 	
Blood Pressure
Palpated
Auscultated
  Location
  Sitting
  Standing
  Lying
		Apical
		
		Systolic
		Systolic/Diastolic
			Peripheral

Analysis:

_____

_____

_____

_____

Pain Assessment

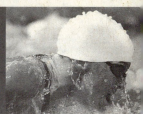

8

OVERVIEW

Pain is subjective. Although we may see the impact of pain, the results of pain, and the sequelae of pain, we will never see pain. Consequently, the nurse must have a sound knowledge about the physiology and treatment of pain and have valid and reliable tools for its assessment. It is the nurse who has the greatest exposure to the client in pain, and so it is the nurse who must be most expert in its assessment. The nurse, in the role of client advocate, is professionally and morally obligated to ensure that clients receive prompt and professional treatment for pain.

ASSIGNMENT

CD-ROM content: Chapter 8
Companion website: www.prenhall.com/damico, Chapter 8

VOCABULARY EXERCISE

After completing the reading assignment, you should be able to define the **key terms** listed below. Refer back to the page number from the main text for help.

Acute pain, 127
Chronic pain, 127
Cutaneous pain, 127
Deep somatic pain, 127
Hyperalgesia, 128
Intractable pain, 127
Neuropathic pain, 127
Nociception, 125
Nociceptors, 125

Pain, 124
Pain reaction, 128
Pain sensation, 128
Pain threshold, 128
Pain tolerance, 128
Phantom pain, 128
Radiating pain, 127
Referred pain, 127
Visceral pain, 127

ANATOMY EXERCISES

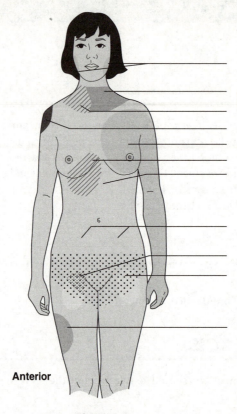

Anterior

Figure 8–1

1. Each shaded area represents a site where organ pain may be referred. Label each area with the organ name. What is the basis for referred pain?

2. Why is this diagram of referred pain sites important knowledge for the nurse?

STUDY FOCUS

1. The concept of specific theory is presented on page 124 of your text. The text informs that this theory does not include a consideration of any psychological component of pain. What impact could psychological factors have? Could there be positive psychological factors for pain?

2. Understanding the physiology of transduction (as explained expertly in the text) assists the nurse in selecting analgesic treatment of pain. What drug is mentioned in this section of Chapter 8, and what is its mechanism of action?

3. What are some advantages of acute pain? What are some disadvantages? Consider concepts presented such as coping, adaptation, and time limitation.

4. A client complaining of pain in the neck could be experiencing what condition(s)?

5. Discuss some reasons why a client may not complain of pain or might refuse treatment of pain when the nurse suspects there is pain present.

REVIEW QUESTIONS

1. The transmission of pain may be interrupted by
   a. CNS sedation.
   b. local anesthetic.
   c. tricyclic antidepressants.
   d. distraction.
   e. all of the above.

2. Factors crucial to assisting the client experiencing pain include

   _____, _____, and _____.

3. Physiological responses to chronic pain are often lessened over time. This is because, over time, the actual pain receptors adapt to the painful stimulus.
   a. true
   b. false

4. Pain experienced by many women at the time of menses may be classified as _____ pain.
   a. referred
   b. visceral
   c. intractable
   d. neuropathic

5. Phantom pain is
   a. emotionally based.
   b. neurogenic in origin.
   c. unrelated to actual pathology.
   d. indicative of damaged stump revision.

6. A client who is excessively sensitive to a particular pain sensation
   a. has a high pain threshold.
   b. is hyperalgesic.
   c. has an unrealistic pain reaction.
   d. is probably attention seeking.

7. Pain control in newborns is poorly understood because it is not clear which neurologic components necessary for pain sensation are present at birth.
   a. true
   b. false

8. Elderly clients may have (circle all that apply)
   a. more than one painful condition.
   b. a pain threshold changed due to aging.
   c. an increased sensitivity to analgesics.
   d. an attitude of inevitability toward pain.

9. The best tool for assessment of pain is (circle all that apply)
    a. the gate control theory.
    b. a focused history.
    c. a unidimensional tool.
    d. a brief pain inventory.
    e. multimodal.

10. List major/common physiological responses seen with acute pain.

11. List as many factors as you can that tend to increase the perception of pain.

CASE STUDY

1. Carl, age 42, arrives in your emergency department complaining of chest pain. When asked to place his hand on the area of greatest pain, he clutches his epigastric area. He is startled looking and appears fearful. His health history is negative for cardiovascular disease. His negative health behaviors include smoking and a moderately sedentary lifestyle. You assess his vital signs as follows:

   Blood pressure 164/94

   Pulse 100

   Respiratory rate 24 and shallow

   Temperature 98.2 oral

   - Given the location indicated, what are some possible reasons for his pain?

   - Are the vital signs given indicative of pain? Are there other possibilities for the vital signs?

   - What is the minimum information you need regarding the pain according to national standards?

   - What are some possible reasons for Carl to be fearful? How would his fear affect his pain perception? Why?

   - Review nursing diagnoses for pain in **Appendix A of your text**.

CLINICAL ACTIVITIES

Using the sample documentation form at the end of the chapter as a guideline, perform a pain assessment on a willing volunteer who can recall a painful experience.

▶ Instruct your volunteer to recall a specific painful experience and to answer your questions in the focused history based on his or her memory of the pain.

▶ Take the focused history as outlined in the guidelines, and add any additional questions needed for clarification.

▶ Provide your volunteer with adequate instruction for the use of the pain scales at the end of this chapter, and ask him or her to indicate the level of pain recalled.

NURSING DIAGNOSES

Select the nursing diagnoses in **Appendix A of your text** that relate directly to pain. Are there any other diagnoses that also reflect a state of pain or discomfort? Remember, the use of pain scales to objectify the nursing diagnoses of pain will improve your ability to treat and monitor your client's condition.

Sample Documentation Form

Guidelines for Pain History	
PAIN HISTORY	
Location	
Onset	
Intensity	
Quality	
Pattern	
Precipitating factors	
Relief/alleviating attempts	Successful?
Impacts on ADL	
Coping strategy	
Emotional response	
Vital signs	Pulse _____ Temp _____ RR _____ BP _____

Pain assessment tool used _____

Sample Documentation Form

Pain Assessment: Tools

Name: _____ Date: _____

Age: _____ Gender: _____

Pain History

    Onset: When did this start? _____

    Location: Where is the pain felt most? Does it radiate? _____
_____

    Intensity: Ask for description. Use the pain scales that follow. _____
_____

    Quality: Is pain sharp, dull, throbbing, etc.? _____
_____

    Pattern: Is the pain intermittent? Constant? Does it wax and wane? _____
_____

    Precipitating factors:
        What seems to bring this pain on? _____
        Noise? _____
        Motion of a body part? _____
        Eating, not eating, etc.? _____

    Relieving factors and attempts to relieve:
        What helps? _____
        Medications? _____
        Heat, ice, etc.? _____

    Impact on activities of daily living: Does this pain prevent usual activities? _____
_____

    Coping strategies (such as prayer, meditation, etc.): _____
_____

    Emotional response (anger, blaming, depression, anxiety, etc.): _____
_____

    Sleep pattern (ability to sleep): _____

    Observation:

    Client behavior (protective posturing, crying, moaning, etc.): _____
_____

    Physiological Responses:

                                       Vital Signs: Temperature: _____

                                              Respirations: _____

                                              Pulse: _____

                                             Blood pressure: _____

Adult Tools

Several visual and verbal tools are available to assess a client's pain. Following are several examples commonly used for the verbal adult. In each case, the client is asked to point along the line to describe the degree of pain.

Visual Analog Scale (VAS)

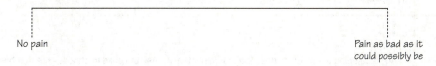

No pain   Pain as bad as it could possibly be

0–10 Numeric Pain Intensity Scale

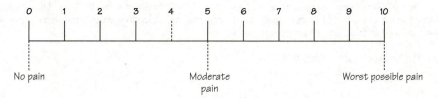

No pain   Moderate pain   Worst possible pain

Simple Descriptive Pain Intensity Scale

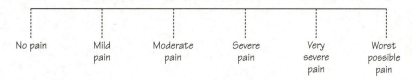

No pain   Mild pain   Moderate pain   Severe pain   Very severe pain   Worst possible pain

Pain Distress Scale

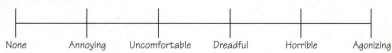

None   Annoying   Uncomfortable   Dreadful   Horrible   Agonizing

Infants and Children

The **OUCHER Pain Scale** is a valid and reliable scale for both young and older children of various races. This scale, is copyrighted and may be purchased for use in the clinical agency. For more information, see, http://www.oucher.org.

Analysis:

_____
_____
_____
_____

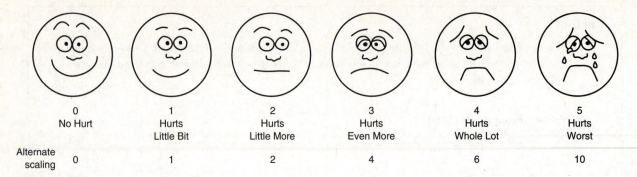

0	1	2	3	4	5
No Hurt	Hurts Little Bit	Hurts Little More	Hurts Even More	Hurts Whole Lot	Hurts Worst

Alternate scaling	0	1	2	4	6	10

Brief word instructions: Point to each face using the words to describe the pain intensity. Ask the child to choose face that best describes own pain and record the appropriate number.

Original instructions: Explain to the person that each face is for a person who feels happy because he has no pain (hurt) or sad because he has some or a lot of pain. Face 0 is very happy because he doesn't hurt at all. Face 1 hurts just a little bit. Face 2 hurts a little more. Face 3 hurts even more. Face 4 hurts a whole lot. Face 5 hurts as much as you can imagine, although you don't have to be crying to feel this bad. Ask the person to choose the face that best describes how he is feeling.

Rating scale is recommended for persons age 3 years and older.

Figure 8–2
Wong-Baker FACES Pain Rating Scale
From Hockenberrry MJ, Wilson D, Winkelstein ML: *Wong's Essentials of Pediatric Nursing*, ed.7 St. Louis, 2005, p. 1259. Used with permission. Copyright, Mosby.

Nutritional Assessment

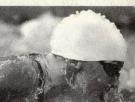

9

OVERVIEW

Nutrition is essential to life, so nutritional assessment is a fundamental part of health assessment. Chapter 9 provides the nurse with a guideline for assessment plus a thorough discussion of the rationale for focus, formulas for anthropometric measurement, and application to health across the life span.

ASSIGNMENT

CD-ROM content: Chapter 9
Companion website: www.prenhall.com/damico, Chapter 9, especially Toolbox

VOCABULARY EXERCISE

After completing the reading assignment, you should be able to define the **key terms** listed below. Refer back to the page number from the main text for help.

Anabolism, 150
Angular stomatitis, 146
Anthropometric, 139
Catabolism, 150
Cheilosis, 146
Diet recall, 138
Flag sign, 146
Food frequency questionnaire, 138
Glossitis, 147
Immunocompetence, 150

Koilonychia, 149
Malnutrition, 136
Overnutrition, 136
Pica, 140
Protein-calorie malnutrition, 136
Rickets, 148
Somatic protein, 13
Undernutrition, 136
Xanthelasma, 146
Xerophthalmia, 146

STUDY FOCUS

1. Which seems to be the more serious problem with malnutrition: undernutrition or overnutrition? Why?

2. What are the outcome measures for nutrition?

3. What are the purposes of anthropometric measurements? Which are the essential measurements for the adult, the infant, and the older adult?

4. Would nutritional deficiencies be entirely dependent on socioeconomic factors?

5. What basic health promotion advice regarding nutrition could a nurse give any adult client?

REVIEW QUESTIONS

1. The four aspects of a nutritional assessment are
   _____, _____, _____, and
   _____ .

2. A diet history that includes recall of food groups rather than specific foods eaten is a
   a. food diary.
   b. food frequency questionnaire.
   c. 24-hour recall.
   d. food pyramid.

3. Appropriate weight for height individualized by formula is
   a. skinfold thickness index.
   b. body mass index.
   c. mid-upper arm circumference.
   d. Metropolitan height-weight table.

4. A BMI of 27 is designated as
   a. overweight.
   b. obese.
   c. mild malnutrition.
   d. normal.

5. Identify factors that would limit the usefulness and validity of a waist circumference measure:
   _____ and _____

6. The skin and mucous membranes are especially vulnerable to which nutritional deficiencies?

CASE STUDY

Mary Smith has brought her two children, ages 4 and 6, in for well-child exams. Both children are in healthy nutritional state, but the 6-year-old will start school this fall. Mrs. Smith wants to know how to manage her family's nutrition proactively. Her husband has a sedentary job. Mrs. Smith says she often has little time to eat during the day, usually finishing whatever the children leave at breakfast and lunch. What advice can you give Mrs. Smith for the adults' and children's calorie and nutrient planning? What resources would you recommend for her reference?

What nursing diagnoses could be appropriate for this client? List as many as seem plausible to you. Discuss with your classmates why you think these diagnoses may be applicable. **See Appendix A in your text** for review of nursing diagnoses.

CLINICAL ACTIVITY

Using the sample documentation form at the end of the chapter as a guideline, perform a nutritional assessment on a willing volunteer, such as your lab partner, roommate, or family member.

▶ Be sure to provide privacy for both the interview and the anthropometric measurements.
▶ Ask about any cultural or religious implications for diet.
▶ Ask about personal taste and habit.

Using the tools in this chapter, perform a nutritional assessment on yourself.

▶ What advice are you ready to give yourself based on derived data?
▶ Do you think you will attempt to take this advice.
▶ How will this experience affect your attitude towards clients?

Refer to Appendix G in your text for the Mini Nutritional Assessment, and use this tool for assessment.

▶ What differences did you find with each tool?
▶ Did you find one more helpful than the other? If so, why?

Sample Documentation Form

GUIDELINES FOR NUTRITION ASSESSMENT

Name: _____ Date: _____

Age: _____ Gender: _____

History

Review of history related to nutrition:

_____

YES/NO			If YES, provide details:

☐ ☐   Recent weight gain   _____

☐ ☐   Recent weight loss   _____

☐ ☐   Concerned about weight   _____

☐ ☐   Dieting at present   _____

☐ ☐   Appetite change   _____

☐ ☐   Food allergies or intolerances   _____

☐ ☐   On special diet at present   _____

☐ ☐   Use of food supplements   _____

☐ ☐   Use of weight-controlling drugs   _____

☐ ☐   Eating disorders   _____

☐ ☐   Experiences of fatigue   _____

☐ ☐   Changes in skin and mucous membranes   _____

Family history of diet, nutrition, or weight problems: _____

_____

_____

Exercise routines: _____

Focused symptom analysis of current nutrition or dietary concern:

Problem statement: _____

     Character: _____

     Onset: _____

     Duration: _____

     Location: _____

     Severity: _____

     Associated problems: _____

     Efforts to treat: _____

Dietary Recall Past 24 Hours

Breakfast: Food: _____

     Portion size: _____

Lunch: Food: _____

     Portion size: _____

Dinner: Food: _____

Portion size: _____

Snacks: Foods: _____

Portion size: _____

Beverages _____

Alcoholic beverages _____

Physical Assessment

Vital Signs

Temperature: _____   Pulse: _____   Respirations: _____   Blood pressure: _____

Inspection of skin and mucous membranes (observe for bruising, poor healing, dryness, poor turgor, cracking):

_____

_____

_____

_____

Inspect the tongue:

_____

Height

Client must remove shoes before evaluating height.

Height in inches: _____ Convert to _____ centimeters; Convert to _____ meters.

[_____ inches $\times$ 2.54 = _____ centimeters]

[_____ centimeters $\times$ 0.1 = _____ meters]

Weight

Time of assessment: _____ a.m. p.m. (circle)

Type of scales being used: ☐ Platform balance beam

☐ Platform digital scale

☐ Bed scale (built into bed)

☐ Swing or chair scale

☐ Floor scale that accommodates wheelchair

Clothing worn by client at time of weighing:

_____

Weight in pounds: _____ Convert to _____ kilograms.

[$\frac{\text{_____ pounds}}{2.2}$ = _____ kilograms]

Physical Measurements

Arm span: _____ inches   _____ centimeters

Mid-arm circumference: _____ inches   _____ centimeters

Triceps circumference: _____ inches   _____ centimeters

Skinfold thickness: Area of body measured _____

_____ inches   _____ centimeters

Body Mass Index

$$\text{Body mass index (BMI)} = \frac{\text{Weight (kg)}}{\text{Height (m)}^2} \text{ or } \frac{\text{weight (lbs)}}{\text{height (inches)}^2} \times 703 = \text{BMI}$$

BMI: 20–24.9, normal

25–29.9, overweight

30 and above, obese

Central Fat Distribution   Waist circumference/Hip circumference = Ratio

Indications of abnormal central fat distribution

Female ratio > 0.8

Male ratio > 9.9

Analysis:

_____

_____

_____

_____

Nutrition Assessment Form

NUTRITION EVALUATION

Name: _____ Date: _____

Home Address: _____ Referred By: _____

_____

Phone: _____

Age: _____ Signed Consent/Date: _____

Height (Ht) _____ Weight (Wt) _____ Recent wt change ____ Max/Min wts _____ Client goal _____

Body fat % _____ Wt Hx _____ Exercise _____ Ex. freq/duration ____ Other activities _____

Medical Hx/Dx _____ Rx and OTC meds ____ Vits/minerals _____ Supplements _____ Herbs _____

Previous Diets _____ Food allergies/   Food prep/refrig _____ Restrictive? _____ Living with _____
                     intolerances _____   Binge? _____

                                                           Purge? _____

                                                        Laxatives? _____

                                                          Other? _____

Diet Hx: _____ Diet Hx: _____

M-F _____ Weekends _____

FOOD FREQUENCY

Fruit (indicate day/week/other)   **Dairy** (indicate day/week/other)   **Fats** (indicate day/week/other)

vit C _____ milk/yogurt _____ saturated _____

other _____ cheese _____ polyunsaturated _____

_____ other _____ monounsaturated _____

Vegetables   **Animal protein**   **Sugars/sweets**

green _____ _____ _____

other _____ _____ _____

Grains/starch   **Plant protein**   **Fluids-water**

whole grain _____ _____ other _____

other _____ _____ caffeinated _____

                                                                                  alcohol

Source: Provided courtesy of Sheila Tucker, MA, RD, LDN.

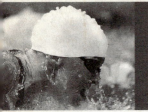

10   The Health History

OVERVIEW

Chapter 10 presents the health history and the interview techniques used in obtaining the data. The health history, as developed by the nurse, is composed of subjective data, is holistic, and is focused on the client. It includes data regarding past and current health as discovered in the interview with the client (if capable), from the medical record, and from caregivers if necessary. Interview techniques used to obtain the history are discussed, and documentation guidelines are given.

ASSIGNMENT

CD-ROM content: Chapter 10
Companion website: www.prenhall.com/damico, Chapter 10

VOCABULARY EXERCISE

After completing the reading assignment, you should be able to define the **key terms** listed below. Refer back to the page number from the main text for help.

Attending, 158	Health pattern, 171
Communication, 157	Interactional skills, 157
Concreteness, 163	Listening, 158
Empathy, 163	Paraphrasing, 158
Encoding, 157	Positive regard, 162
False reassurance, 160	Preinteraction phase, 164
Focused interview, 166	Primary source, 170
Genogram, 173	Reflecting, 159
Genuineness, 163	Secondary source, 164
Health history, 151	Summarizing, 160

STUDY FOCUS

1. What are the components of a communication process? Give an example of something that can hamper communication through each of its processes.

2. There are a variety of question formats. List three and give an example of each, indicating when each type would be most appropriate in a specific situation.

3. What is the difference between a primary and a secondary source for historical information? When would it be appropriate to use a secondary source?

4. What aspects of health would be affected by cultural factors? How would the nature of a role be affected by cultural factors?

REVIEW QUESTIONS

1. When you want to encourage your clients to explore or generally discuss their impression of their health, the following type of question is most useful.
   a. Open-ended question
   b. closed question
   c. limit setting
   d. reflecting

2. As the history-taking phase of the nurse-client encounter comes to an end, the following technique used by the nurse will assist both the client and the nurse to ensure that no data is omitted and that the two share a common understanding.
   a. focusing
   b. attending
   c. questioning
   d. summarizing

3. Your client's chief complaint is "I've had this irritating cough for a week." As you spend the next 12 minutes gathering pertinent data in the interview, you notice that you do not observe him coughing, and so you share this observation with him. You are
   a. rude.
   b. distracting.
   c. attending.
   d. reflecting.

4. You are caring for a client who admits to postoperative pain, yet refuses pain-relieving medication. This client behavior could indicate
   a. a cultural belief in the acceptance of pain as trial or punishment.
   b. fear of medications.
   c. client belief in alternative therapy.
   d. any of the above.

5. Which of the following is essential to every client interview?
   a. courtesy
   b. open-ended questions
   c. family history
   d. reflection techniques

6. Which statement is correct concerning information pertinent to a history? Information should be
   a. shared with the family only at the discretion of the nurse.
   b. specific as to race and culture.
   c. generalized as to culture.
   d. all of the above.

7. The history of the present illness is
   a. body system interaction with the chief complaint.
   b. circumstances surrounding the chief complaint.
   c. detailed discussion of any associated factors of the chief complaint.
   d. all of the above.

8. When taking a history, you should
   a. start the interview with the client's identifying data.
   b. use a chronological and sequential framework.
   c. clarify any broad statements.
   d. all of the above.

9. Your client mentions his use of alcohol and illicit drugs. This information would most likely belong in the
   a. chief complaint.
   b. past medical history.
   c. psychosocial history.
   d. review of systems.

10. Seeking clarification through questioning is a direct verbal technique that can assist the nurse to gather accurate data during
    a. physical assessment.
    b. history taking.
    c. interpretation of body language.
    d. interpretation of medical records.
    e. all of the above.

SITUATION

Your client tells you, the nurse, that she must confer with her mother-in-law before accepting a clearly needed medical procedure. You defer to her wishes but privately think her behavior is irrational and dangerous.

11. You are demonstrating _____ in your behavior.
    a. cultural acceptance
    b. ethnocentrism
    c. cultural shock
    d. cultural relativism

12. But you are demonstrating _____ in your thinking.
    a. cultural acceptance
    b. ethnocentrism
    c. cultural shock
    d. cultural relativism

13. All of the following are primary (firsthand) sources of data the nurse can use to gather information about the client *except*
    a. the interview process.
    b. the physical assessment.
    c. the client's significant others.
    d. direct observations of the client's behavior.

14. An important component of the nursing assessment is the medical history. An example of the past medical history data you would gather is
    a. the client's previous hospitalizations, surgeries, and illnesses.
    b. causes of death in the client's close family members.
    c. the client's present symptoms and concerns.
    d. review of current laboratory tests performed on the client.

15. The client tells the nurse that he has recently experienced a loss of appetite. This represents which kind of data?
    a. nutritional
    b. secondary
    c. subjective
    d. objective

16. Which of the following techniques is most likely to result in the client's understanding of questions?
    a. Use phrases that are commonly used by other clients in the area.
    b. Use the client's own terms whenever possible.
    c. Use only medical and technical terminology.

17. When you question a client regarding alcohol intake, she tells you that she is "only a social drinker." Which initial response is appropriate?
    a. "I'm glad that you are a responsible drinker."
    b. "Do the other people in your household consume alcohol?"
    c. "What amount and what kind of alcohol do you drink in a week?"
    d. "If you only drink socially, you won't need to worry about always having a designated driver."

CASE STUDY

1. You are admitting Reba, a 17-year-old, to your medical-surgical unit. She tells you that she is Catholic, the oldest of three sisters, and a full-time student. Reba mentions that she is a member of her high school pep squad and has injured her ankle dancing. She has never been in a hospital as a patient so there are no medical records available for review. Her mother is with her, and there is the possibility of a surgical repair of her ankle.

   • As you take a complete health history, what areas will become especially important? Why?

   • Will you implement the interview with or without the presence of her mother?

- What developmental considerations may be important with this client?

- What might be the areas for a more focused history, within the complete history?

CLINICAL ACTIVITIES

Create a genogram of your family with you as the primary client. What patterns do you see?

Using the sample documentation form at the end of this chapter as a guideline, take a complete health history from someone who agrees to give you adequate time and attention.

▶ Even though this is a practice history, the rules of privacy and confidentiality remain the same.

▶ Be careful with what becomes of this document after your practice and a possible review by your instructor as it will not become a medical record. Be sure to dispose of it very carefully.

Note how the Mini Nutritional History (**Appendix G in your text**) may be a useful part of the history.

Sample Documentation Form

Complete Health History

Name: _____ Date: _____

Age: _____ Gender: _____ Marital Status: _____ Race: _____ Ethnicity: _____

Culture: _____ Religion: _____ Occupation: _____

Health Insurance: _____ Source of Information/Reliability: _____

Date of Last Visit:

History

Review of history related to the reason for the client's visit:

Focused symptom analysis of current problem:

    Reason for seeking healthcare: _____

    _____

    Description of present problem:

    Onset: _____

    Duration: _____

    Location: _____

    Severity: _____

    Associated problems: _____

    Efforts to treat: _____

Health beliefs and practices: _____

_____

_____

Health patterns/general health status: _____

Sleep/rest/stress-reduction patterns: _____

_____

Current medications (Rx, OTC, complementary): _____

_____

_____

_____

Allergies: _____

_____

Past Medical History

    Past medical problems: _____

    _____

    _____

    Hospitalizations and surgery: _____

Primary care: _____

_____

_____

Childhood illnesses: _____

_____

_____

Immunizations: _____

_____

Mental and emotional health: _____

_____

Substance use: _____

Family History

Immediate family: _____

Extended family: _____

Genogram:

Psychosocial History

Occupational history: _____

Education: _____

Financial background:

_____

Roles and independence: _____

_____

Family: _____

Social structure: _____

Emotional concerns: _____

Self-concept: _____

Current Medical History/Review of Systems

_____

YES/NO	If YES, provide details:

Review of Systems

☐ ☐ Nutrition   _____

_____

☐ ☐ Hair, skin, nails   _____

_____

☐ ☐ Head and neck   _____

_____

☐ ☐ Lymphatics   _____

_____

☐ ☐ Eyes/vision _____

☐ ☐ Ears/hearing _____

☐ ☐ Nose, mouth, throat _____

☐ ☐ Respiratory system _____

☐ ☐ Cardiovascular _____

☐ ☐ Circulatory or peripheral vascular _____

☐ ☐ Breasts and axillae _____
☐ ☐ Abdomen/gastrointestinal _____

☐ ☐ Musculoskeletal _____

☐ ☐ Neurologic _____

☐ ☐ Female reproductive _____
☐ ☐ Male reproductive
☐ ☐ Mental health
☐ ☐ Rectal, bowels, prostate _____

Analysis:

_____

_____

_____

_____

Skin, Hair, and Nails 11

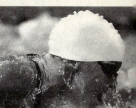

OVERVIEW

The integumentary system is the largest (and heaviest) system of the body. It reflects nutritional status, circulatory and pulmonary status, and its own development and maintenance integrity. Adventitious findings in this system may indicate primary integumentary problems or be reflections of disturbances in other systems. Assessment of this system yields a wide range of information and clues to the general health of the entire client.

ASSIGNMENT

CD-ROM content: Chapter 11
Companion website: www.prenhall.com/damico, Chapter 11

VOCABULARY EXERCISE

After completing the reading assignment, you should be able to define the **key terms** listed below. Refer back to the page number from the main text for help.

Alopecia, 206
Apocrine glands, 184
Chloasma, 187
Cuticle, 185
Dandruff, 206
Dermis, 183
Diaphoresis, 203
Ecchymosis, 204
Eccrine glands, 184
Edema, 204
Epidermis, 183
Hair, 185
Hypodermis, 184
Keratin, 183
Lanugo, 186
Linea nigra, 187

Lunula, 185
Melanin, 183
Milia, 186
Mongolian spots, 186
Nails, 185
Onycholysis, 208
Paronychia, 208
Pediculosis capitis, 207
Primary lesions, 204
Pruritus, 195
Sebaceous glands, 184
Secondary lesions, 204
Terminal hair, 185
Vellus hair, 185
Vernix caseosa, 186
Vitiligo, 202

ANATOMY EXERCISES

1. Label hair shaft, oil gland, eccrine glands, epidermis, dermis, and subcutaneous tissue.

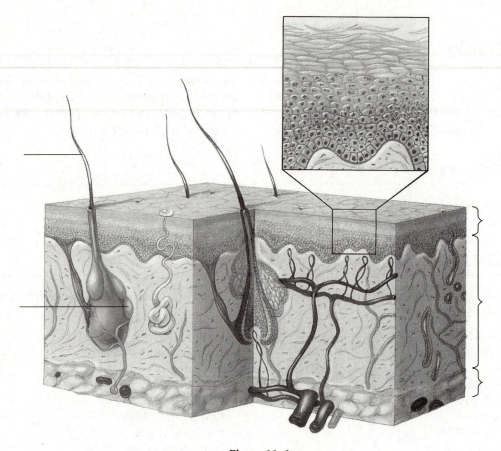

Figure 11–1

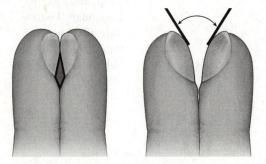

Figure 11–2

2. Which is the expected finding? What chronic condition can result in this finding of clubbing?

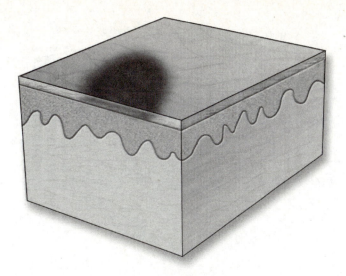

Figure 11–3

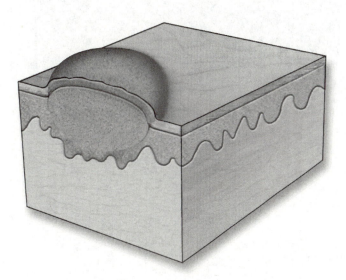

Figure 11–4

3. Give examples of macules and papules.

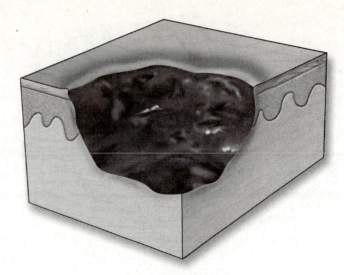

Figure 11–5

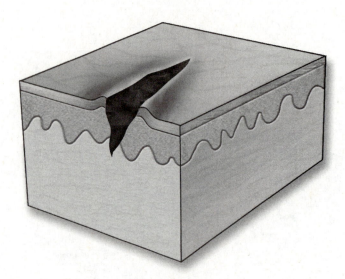

Figure 11–6

4. Give examples of fissures and ulcers.

5. What layers of tissue are involved in an ulcer?

6. What layers are involved in a fissure?

STUDY FOCUS

1. Describe what you would find on a general survey of the skin. Remember that a general survey uses only the technique of inspection. List at least four characteristics you can identify in this manner.

2. What characteristics of the skin require the technique of palpation? List at least four.

3. How does the normal skin of the aging adult compare to the normal skin of a younger adult or adolescent?

4. What are the documentation standards for describing a lesion?

REVIEW QUESTIONS

1. While all are important, one of the most critical general historical questions for integumentary relating to health promotion is about
   a. vitamin C intake.
   b. amount of ultraviolet ray exposure.
   c. skin breaks.
   d. use of specific hygiene products.

Matching: Indicate which of the terms pertaining to skin color matches each of the following.
   a. albinism
   b. jaundice
   c. carotenemia
   d. cyanosis

2. decreased oxygenation _____

3. increased level of bilirubin _____

4. generalized lack of color _____

5. Tangential lighting is most important for inspecting skin
   a. color.
   b. contour/lesions.
   c. exudates.
   d. symmetry.
   e. a and b.

6. A slightly elevated brownish papule with indistinct borders is a typical characteristic of
   a. nevus.
   b. petechiae.
   c. papule.
   d. vesicle.

7. Lesions that are arranged in a circular pattern are
   a. irregular.
   b. annular.
   c. stellate.
   d. reticulate.

8. The most common cutaneous neoplasm is
   a. basal cell carcinoma.
   b. nevus.
   c. seborrheic keratosis.
   d. senile actinic keratosis.

Matching: Indicate which description matches each of the following.
   a. raised
   b. fluid filled
   c. round
   d. fluid to semisolid filled
   e. localized edema

9. macule _____

10. vesicle _____

11. bullous _____

12. cyst _____

13. Thick toughened layers of skin are called
   a. desquamation.
   b. scaling.
   c. lichenification.
   d. crust.

14. A linear crack in the epidermis, sometimes to the dermis, is
   a. erosion.
   b. an ulcer.
   c. a fissure.
   d. excoriation.

15. Inspection of fingernails can yield information relative to
   a. nutritional status.
   b. oxygenation.
   c. infection.
   d. all of the above.

16. Due to the increased pigmentation of skin during pregnancy, _____ is a common and benign finding in a pregnant woman.
   a. hemangioma
   b. linea nigra
   c. chloasma
   d. vitiligo
   e. b and c

17. Common findings on the skin of a term infant include
   a. lanugo.
   b. cutaneous horn.
   c. ecchymosis.
   d. vernix caseosa.
   e. a and d.

18. Distribution of skin lesions that are clearly defined and separate is referred to as _____, while lesions that overlap and flow together indistinctly are referred to as _____.
   a. macular, patches
   b. stellate, annular
   c. discrete, confluent
   d. lesions, coloration

19. Older adults tend to have _____ compared to younger adults and children.
   a. more subcutaneous tissue
   b. less subcutaneous tissue

CASE STUDIES

1. Beth, a first-time mother, brings in 6-week-old Michael for a well-child checkup. Beth is fairly distressed over the many skin imperfections she has found on her little son. There are, according to Beth's report, red blotches everywhere, tiny white pimples on his face, and hair on his back. Beth asks if this is because she had skin changes during pregnancy resulting in dark nipples, a brown line down her stomach, and a shadow over the bridge of her nose. She asks if Michael's skin problems will require treatment and if they can be cured.

   ● What health history questions are especially important for mother and baby?

   ● When would client teaching be most effective—before or after the physical examination? Why?

   ● What do you suspect is the logical explanation for the complaints about baby's skin?

   ● What is the logical explanation for the complaints about mother's skin?

   ● What should be documented about skin on the baby's medical record?

2. Jack, age 72, is being seen for the removal of some suspicious skin lesions. As you take admitting information, Jack says he is not worried about the procedure. "I guess everyone has to die of something," he says briskly.

- What kind of reassurance can you properly give Jack before the procedure and its results?

- What should your focused interview questions reveal?

- Should you do a skin assessment or assume that would be redundant given that lesions have already been identified?

- What might you anticipate given Jack's expected healing course after the procedure?

- What nursing diagnoses would be applicable to Jack's situation? **See Appendix A in your text** to review diagnoses as needed.

CLINICAL ACTIVITIES

Using the sample documentation form at the end of the chapter as a guideline, perform a skin assessment on your lab partner or a willing volunteer. Skin assessment may be done as a separate system or integrated into the head-to-toe exam where the skin is assessed as the exam proceeds from area to area.

▸ Take a history, focusing on any areas of concern for the client, and then prepare to do a physical assessment.
▸ Review the advice in your text for beginning assessment of the skin.
▸ Have equipment, gown, drapes, gloves, lighting, and ruler ready and ensure privacy for your client during the history and assessment.

▸ Remember that you must protect yourself from exposure to any blood or body fluids, and your client from contaminated equipment. **Please see Appendices B and C in your text** to review protective measures for the nurse and equipment.

During an actual physical assessment with a client, this is an opportune time to teach techniques of skin assessment and the importance of skin self-exam. Suggest ways for the client to remember to examine the skin, such as once a month on a birth date, or when the client pays a monthly bill.

Sample Documentation Form for Assessment

Skin, Hair, and Nails

Name: _____ Date: _____

Age: _____ Gender: _____

History

Review of history related to hair, skin, and nails:

YES/NO		If YES, provide details:

General

☐	☐	Current integumentary problems	_____
☐	☐	Illness during past week	_____
☐	☐	Current medical conditions	_____
☐	☐	Change in color or texture of skin	_____
☐	☐	Allergies	_____

Skin

☐	☐	Dry or oily skin	_____
☐	☐	Current skin condition	_____
☐	☐	Lesions or infections	_____
☐	☐	Pain or itching of skin	_____
☐	☐	Scales, scabs, or flaking	_____
☐	☐	Body odor	_____
☐	☐	Recent or increased bruising	_____
☐	☐	Change in mole	_____
☐	☐	Sores that do not heal	_____
☐	☐	History of skin cancer	_____
☐	☐	Usual sun exposure	_____
☐	☐	Use of sunscreen	_____
☐	☐	Occupational exposures	_____

Hair

☐	☐	Changes in hair texture	_____
☐	☐	Changes in hair amount	_____
☐	☐	Scalp irritation or itching	_____
☐	☐	Scalp infection or infestation	_____
☐	☐	Use of dyes or bleach	_____

Nails

☐	☐	Problems or changes in nails	_____
☐	☐	Increased brittleness	_____
☐	☐	Color or shape changes	_____
☐	☐	Infections of the nails	_____
☐	☐	Wear artificial nails	_____
☐	☐	Biting or chewing nails	_____

Family history of problems relating to the skin, hair, and nails: _____
_____

Review of history related to the current visit:

Reason for visit:_____
_____

Focused symptom analysis of current problem:

Character: _____

Onset: _____

Duration: _____

Location: _____

Severity: _____

Associated problems: _____

Efforts to treat: _____

Current medications: _____
_____
_____

Allergies: _____
_____

Physical Assessment

Ensure overhead and moveable light sources are working. Have client disrobed and draped for privacy.
Ensure warmth of room. Have gloves available to the nurse.

Skin:

Inspect and palpate the skin.

General appearance (cleanliness, color, evenness of color/pigmentation, texture, moisture, temperature,
edema, intactness, lesions or scars): _____

Body odor: _____

Lesion evaluation: Location: _____

Distribution: _____

Shape: _____

Sizes: _____

Color, texture, distribution: _____

Discharge or exudate (describe): _____

Palpation characteristics: _____

YES	NO		
☐	☐	Infection noted	_____
☐	☐	Infestation	_____
☐	☐	Discolorations	_____

Hair:

Inspect and palpate the hair.

General characteristics—head (color, amount, distribution, texture, moisture):

_____

_____

General characteristics—face, eyebrows (color, amount, distribution, texture, moisture):

_____

_____

General characteristics—body hair (color, amount, distribution, texture, moisture):

_____

_____

YES	NO	
☐	☐	Balding areas _____
☐	☐	Nits or infestations _____

Nails:

Inspect and palpate the nails.

General characteristics—hands (color, texture, grooming, artificial nails, evidence of infection):

_____

_____

General characteristics—feet (color, texture, grooming, evidence of infection):

_____

_____

YES	NO	
☐	☐	Nail clubbing _____
☐	☐	Nail spooning _____
☐	☐	Infection noted _____
☐	☐	Other noted problem _____

Analysis:

_____

_____

_____

_____

_____

Head, Neck, and Related Lymphatics 12

OVERVIEW

Assessment of the head, neck, and related lymphatics encompasses several overlapping systems. It is really the assessment of a region containing critically important systems for health functioning and well-being. History and physical assessment must include aspects of all these systems: skin, neurologic, cardiovascular, musculoskeletal, and immune. The assessment focuses on the integration of sensory, motor, and body defenses.

ASSIGNMENT

CD-ROM content: Chapter 12
Companion website: www.prenhall.com/damico, Chapter 12

VOCABULARY EXERCISE

After completing the reading assignment, you should be able to define the **key terms** listed below. Refer back to the page number from the main text for help.

Acromegaly, 255
Anterior triangle, 237
Atlas, 236
Axis, 236
Bell's palsy, 255
Goiter, 241
Hydrocephalus, 254
Hyoid, 237

Hyperthyroidism, 250
Hypothyroidism, 258
Lymphadenopathy, 252
Posterior triangle, 237
Sutures, 235
Thyroid gland, 237
Torticollis, 257

ANATOMY EXERCISES

1. Label the structures of the neck, when you palpate the thyroid. Note that you can only reach the edges and the anterior surface.

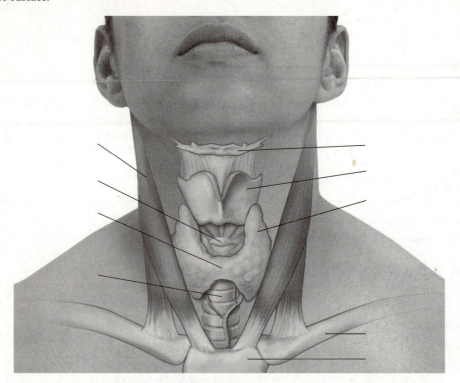

Figure 12–1

2. Label the neck vessels and the sternomastoid muscle.

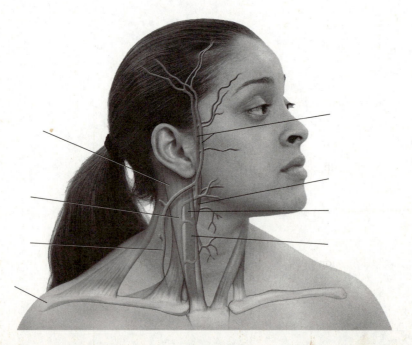

Figure 12–2

3. How will you differentiate the carotid artery from the jugular vein?

4. Indicate the area where you would auscultate the temporal and the carotid arteries.

5. Label the lymphatics of the head and neck.

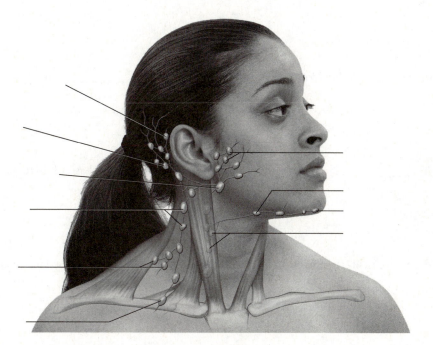

Figure 12–3

6. Which nodes would drain the conjunctiva? Which would drain nasal and sinus areas?

STUDY FOCUS

1. What focused interview findings relating to the client's head would give cause for special physical assessment focus?

2. What are the essential questions to ask of a client giving a history of head injury?

3. How might a pain scale be helpful in documenting a headache?

4. Which systems must be evaluated in the basic inspection of the face?

5. Which significant cardiovascular structures must be evaluated during head and neck assessment?

6. Range of motion of the neck should include _____, _____, _____, and _____.

7. Techniques of _____ and _____ and a focused interview form the basis of thyroid assessment.

8. The head and neck are richly supplied with lymphatics. These nodes should be assessed for what characteristics?

9. Migraine and cluster headaches are vascular headaches by type. What are their commonalities? What are their differences?

REVIEW QUESTIONS

1. Your client gives history of head injury during a routine physical. Which of the following questions yield essential assessment information?
   a. Are there continuing headaches?
   b. How did the injury occur?
   c. Was there loss of consciousness?
   d. Does the client experience seizures?
   e. all of the above

2. *Routine* techniques used to assess the thyroid are
   a. inspection and palpation.
   b. inspection and auscultation.
   c. palpation and lab analysis.
   d. all of the above.

3. A 2-cm nodule on the posterior aspect of the thyroid gland is discernible by
   a. inspection.
   b. palpation.
   c. percussion.
   d. auscultation.
   e. none of the above.

4. Examination of the neck includes (at least partial) evaluation of which of the following systems?
   a. musculoskeletal
   b. lymphatic, skin, cardiovascular
   c. renal, mental
   d. musculoskeletal, endocrine
   e. b and d

5. Shape of the head and proportion of the face is primarily
   a. a cultural influence.
   b. a cosmetic concern.
   c. an indicator of symmetry in growth.
   d. of concern only in children.

6. What data are likely to be pertinent to the history of a woman with a possible thyroid problem?
   a. change in menstrual flow (amount) or frequency
   b. evidence of seizures
   c. increase in lacrimation
   d. presence of varicosities

7. Specific equipment for *routine* examination of the lymphatic system includes a
   a. supply of gloves.
   b. centimeter ruler.
   c. goniometer.
   d. syringe and needle.

8. A child with head lice who has been scratching her scalp aggressively may present with swollen and tender
   a. preauricular nodes.
   b. supraclavicular nodes.
   c. occipital nodes.
   d. epitrochlear nodes.

9. Your client has developed an infection in a blister on her toe. Likely, her _____ node will be enlarged or even tender.
   a. cervical
   b. popliteal
   c. mediastinal
   d. inguinal

10. Historical complaints related to the lymphatic system would include
    a. repeated infections.
    b. swelling of extremities.
    c. easy bruising.
    d. frequent nose/gum bleeds.
    e. all of the above.

11. Among the following findings in evaluation of a lymph node, which is the most ominous (gives cause for greatest concern)?
    a. enlargement
    b. firmness
    c. fixation to underlying tissue
    d. redness
    e. warmth

12. An enlargement or swelling of a lymph node can indicate
    a. infection in a region drained by the node.
    b. a malignant tumor.
    c. allergic responses.
    d. infiltration by foreign substances.
    e. all/any of the above.

13. A headache that presents frequently with bilateral, slow onset of steady pain and is relieved by sleep or moderate exercise is likely a _____ headache.
    a. tension
    b. cluster
    c. PMS
    d. migraine

14. In Bell's palsy, the _____ cranial nerve is affected, resulting in a facial hemiparalysis.

15. The following chronic illness(es) has(have) special facial configurations that help identify its presence:
    a. Cushing syndrome
    b. Down syndrome
    c. hypothyroidism
    d. fetal alcohol syndrome
    e. all of the above

16. Assessment of the head of an infant should include (circle all that apply)
    a. family and birth history.
    b. dietary history.
    c. biparietal measurement.
    d. chest measurement.
    e. headache history.
    f. measurement of fontanels.
    g. facial symmetry.

17. Assessment of the head of a pregnant woman should include especially (circle all that apply and prioritize 1 through 4)
    a. headache history.
    b. history of seizure.
    c. facial edema.
    d. dizziness.

18. List possible head and neck changes in the older adult that would be within normal limits.

Matching:

19. acromegaly _____

20. craniostenosis _____

21. hypothyroidism _____

22. hyperthyroidism _____

23. torticollis _____

24. lymphadenopathy _____

a. unilateral neck muscle spasm
b. misshapen cranium
c. excessive secretion of growth hormone
d. edematous facial features, thickened skin
e. enlarged lymph nodes
f. exophthalmos, startled appearance

25. List health promotion behaviors for healthy adults that are critical to head and neck health.

CASE STUDIES

1. Nancy is a 28-year-old secretary who presents at a primary care practice complaining of frequent and persistent headache. She asks several times during the interview if she might have a brain tumor. She is healthy and her diet is well-balanced. She participates in light physical exercise less than two times monthly.

- List the critical questions for a focused interview.

- What aspects of a general health history would be important?

- What aspects of health promotion would be important for Nancy?

- What nursing diagnoses would be possible for Nancy's concerns?

2. Jean is a 78-year-old retired teacher who is being admitted to the orthopedic unit of your hospital for cervical stabilization. She says that she has had worsening decreased range of motion of her neck for some time. She also has recently noticed some numbness and tingling in her hands.

- List the critical questions for a focused interview.

- What information do you need to plan immediate care for Jean regarding pain control and safety?

- What psychosocial information do you need to plan for Jean's aftercare?

- What nursing diagnoses would be likely for Jean immediately postoperatively?

- What nursing diagnoses would be likely as she recovers at home?

CLINICAL ACTIVITIES

Assessment of the head and neck varies considerably with age of the client, though there are absolutes that must be addressed with clients of all ages. Using the guidelines provided at the end of this chapter:

► Perform a complete assessment of the head, neck, and lymphatics of your lab partner or willing volunteer.
► Review the advice in your text for preparation of equipment, the nurse, and the client for this exam.
► Use the guidelines as only guidelines, pursuing any interesting facts as necessary.

► If your client admits to headaches, be sure to take a complete focused history of the headaches and a pain assessment of the discomfort.

Be sure to protect yourself with gloves, mask, goggles, and any other needed equipment if the client is coughing, is sneezing, or has any discharge with which you might come in contact. Review **Appendices B and C in your text** for appropriate precautions.

Sample Documentation Form

Head, Neck, Thyroid, and Lymphatics

Name: _____ Date: _____

Age: _____ Gender: _____

History

Review of history related to head, neck, thyroid, and lymphatics:

_____

YES/NO   If YES, provide details:

_____

Head, Hair, Scalp, Face

☐ ☐   Head injury   _____
☐ ☐   Headache   _____
☐ ☐   Dizziness/LOC   _____
☐ ☐   Hair problems/loss   _____
☐ ☐   Itching or flaking scalp _____
☐ ☐   Scalp infection/lesions _____
☐ ☐   Facial weakness, swelling _____
☐ ☐   Facial pain or numbness _____

Neck, Thyroid

☐ ☐   History of neck injury   _____
☐ ☐   Neck pain, limitation of motion _____
☐ ☐   Lumps or swelling   _____
☐ ☐   Problems swallowing   _____
☐ ☐   Lump or thickness in throat   _____
☐ ☐   History of thyroid problems   _____
☐ ☐   Fatigue or anxiety   _____
☐ ☐   Weight change   _____

Lymphatics

☐ ☐   Swelling, pain in nodes   _____
☐ ☐   Repeated infections   _____
☐ ☐   Cough or cold   _____
☐ ☐   Recent illness or injury _____
☐ ☐   Allergies   _____

Current medications: _____

Family history of problems relating to hair, scalp, face, lymphatic, or thyroid: _____

_____

Focused symptom analysis of current problem:

   Reason for visit: _____

   _____

   Character: _____

   Onset: _____

   Duration: _____

Location: _____

Severity: _____

Associated problems: _____

Efforts to treat: _____

Physical Assessment

Inspection

    Hair (hair pattern, loss, texture, quantity, quality): _____

_____

    Scalp (intactness, lesions, scars): _____

_____

    Face (color, symmetry, features, lesions, scars, symmetrical mobility): _____

_____

    Eyes (pronounced eyes, wide eye opening, staring appearance): _____

_____

    Temporal, carotid artery (noted distention or pulsations): _____

_____

    Thyroid (swelling, displaced trachea, neck movement limitation): _____

_____

    Lymphatics (node swelling, redness): _____

    Trachea placement: _____

Palpation

    Hair and scalp (hair texture, lesions, pain, tenderness, masses, texture): _____

_____

    Face (pain or tenderness, nodules or swelling, skin texture): _____

_____

    Temporal, carotid artery (pulse rate and quality): _____

_____

    Thyroid (size, symmetry, position, movement with swallowing): _____

_____

    Lymphatics (swelling, warmth, tenderness): _____

    Trachea (mobility, placement): _____

Auscultation

    Temporal arteries (rate, rhythm, bruits): _____

_____

    Carotid arteries (rate, rhythm, bruits): _____

    Thyroid gland (if enlarged): _____

_____

Analysis:

_____

_____

_____

_____

13 Eye

OVERVIEW

Few things are more precious to most of us than our eyes and vision. Assessment of these structures and their functionality is of great importance. Today, there are sound recommendations for health promotion behaviors that are integral to protecting and preserving vision. Obtaining objective and subjective data while maintaining the health of the eyes with client teaching is an important aspect of the role of the professional nurse. Chapter 13 will prepare you to do both.

ASSIGNMENT

CD-ROM content: Chapter 13
Companion website: www.prenhall.com/damico, Chapter 13

VOCABULARY EXERCISE

After completing the reading assignment, you should be able to define the **key terms** listed below. Refer back to the page number from the main text for help.

Accommodation, 282
Aqueous humor, 265
Astigmatism, 290
Blepharitis, 295
Cataract, 269
Choroid, 264
Consensual constriction, 281
Convergence, 282
Cornea, 264
Ectropion, 296
Emmetropia, 265
Entropion, 297
Esophoria, 292
Exophoria, 292
Fundus, 285
Hyperopia, 265
Iris, 264
Iritis, 297

Lens, 265
Macula, 265
Miosis, 264
Mydriasis, 264
Myopia, 265
Nystagmus, 280
Optic disc, 265
Palpebrae, 266
Palpebral fissure, 266
Periorbital edema, 298
Presbyopia, 268
Ptosis, 283
Retina, 265
Sclera, 264
Strabismus, 291
Vitreous humor, 265
Visual field, 290

ANATOMY EXERCISES

1. Label the external eye structures.

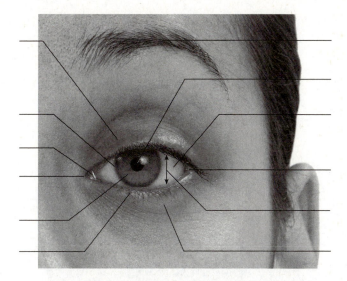

Figure 13–1 External Eye and Lids

2. Indicate where one might find hordeolum and chalazion.

3. Label the structures of the eyeball.

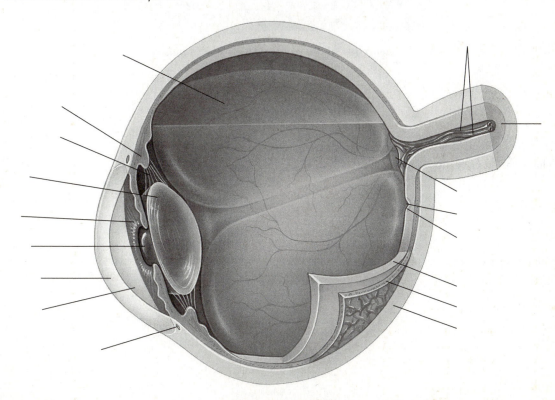

Figure 13–2 Eyeball

4. Indicate where increased pressure associated with glaucoma would occur.

5. Label the eyeball.

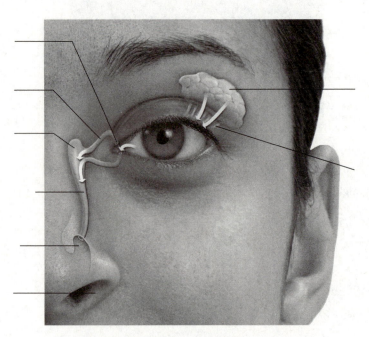

Figure 13–3 Nasolacrimal Ducts and Glands

6. What signs on inspection would indicate a blocked lacrimal duct?

7. Often when we cry we can taste tears. Can you explain this on the basis of this anatomy?

8. Label the six rectus muscles of the eye and the optic nerve.

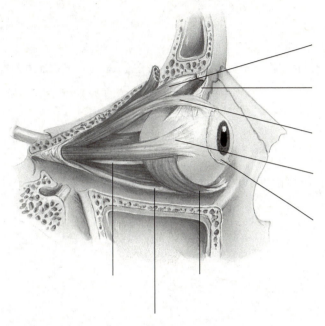

Figure 13–4 Extraocular Muscles

9. What signs are apparent to the examiner when the extraocular muscles of the eye are not in balance with each other? What physical assessment techniques are used to identify these signs?

STUDY FOCUS

1. List health promotion behaviors directed toward eye health that the nurse can address in the focused interview.

2. What structural features of the eye can give clues to possible abnormal conditions?

3. What health history facts could be relevant in a client who reports having "a few" cases of conjunctivitis?

4. Why might it be that a client does not report a vision problem and yet gives positive history for difficulty seeing at either close or far range?

5. Testing vision regularly in the schools is a standard. Now that you've read Chapter 13, do you believe the standard testing to be adequate?

6. What value would there be in performing a funduscopic exam in a primary care setting absent client complaint of eye or vision problem?

REVIEW QUESTIONS

1. Routine techniques of examination relevant to assessment of the eye include
   a. inspection and percussion.
   b. inspection and palpation.
   c. palpation.
   d. auscultation.
   e. inspection.

2. Physical assessment of the eye should proceed from _____ to _____ and from _____ to _____. Choose a or b.
   a. internal, external; specific, general
   b. general, specific; external, internal

3. Snellen's fractions portray vision evaluation in which the _____ indicates the client's distance from the eye chart, and the _____ indicates the distance at which the normal eye could read the chart.
   a. denominator; numerator
   b. numerator; denominator

4. The cover-uncover eye test is important because it is
   a. instrumental in detecting amblyopia.
   b. noninvasive.
   c. capable of testing cranial nerve II.
   d. an evaluation of muscle balance of each eye.
   e. a and d.

5. The conjunctiva is expected to be clear and translucent. Which of the following would be normal findings?
   a. small discrete blood vessels
   b. moderate injection
   c. pink, grainy appearance
   d. profuse clear watery discharge

6. The erythema of conjunctivitis builds from the _____ to the _____ of the eye.

7. The erythema of iritis (infection) builds from the _____ to the _____ of the eye. Choose a or b.
   a. center, periphery
   b. periphery, center

8. Your assessment of Ms. Baker, who states that she is not able to see as clearly in her right eye as she has in the past, should include questions about this symptom such as
   a. decreased moisture.
   b. eye pain.
   c. stress or lack of sleep.
   d. if it is sudden or gradual in onset.
   e. b and d.

9. When examining the lacrimal apparatus, the portion that is actually directly seen is the
   a. lacrimal gland.
   b. lacrimal sac.
   c. nasolacrimal puncta.

10. A pterygium of the bulbar conjunctiva is
    a. a sign of allergic conjunctivitis.
    b. treated with antibiotics.
    c. benign unless it overrides the pupil.
    d. associated with myopia.

11. A bacterial (usually staph or strep) infection of the lid margin that is localized to a single lesion is
    a. blepharitis.
    b. a chalazion.
    c. a hordeolum.
    d. xanthelasma.

Matching:

12. permanent loss of vision _____

13. distance refractive vision error _____

14. protrusion of eye from the socket _____

15. drooping of the lid _____

   a. anisocoria
   b. amblyopia
   c. hyperopia
   d. ptosis
   e. exophthalmos

16. Given the normal eye of client and examiner, you are holding the ophthalmoscope approximately 10 to 12 inches from your client's eye. You want to examine for the red light reflex and the fundus. The best setting of the lens wheel would be
    a. −10 to −15.
    b. −3.
    c. 0.
    d. +2 to +5.
    e. +15 to +20.

17. The physiological eye accommodates to
    a. light.
    b. distant focus.
    c. near focus.
    d. all of the above.

18. Measurement of near vision should be tested
    a. in each eye separately.
    b. with the head at a 45-degree angle.
    c. with the use of primary colors.
    d. using the Snellen chart.

19. Mr. Clinton's visual acuity is 20/50. This means that
    a. he can see 50% of what the average person sees at 20 ft.
    b. he has perfect vision when tested at 50 ft.
    c. he can see 20% of the letters on the chart's 20/50 line.
    d. he can read letters while standing 20 ft from the chart that the average person could read at 50 ft.

20. Findings that can indicate a cataract include
    a. diminished red light reflex.
    b. tiny dark lesions on the macula.
    c. arterio-venous nicking in the fundus.
    d. dull appearance of the pupil on light illumination.
    e. a and d.

21. Observing symmetrical bilateral corneal light reflex is especially important in children and is an evaluation of
    a. corneal sensitivity.
    b. extraocular muscle balance.
    c. PERRLA.
    d. blink response.

SITUATION

Positioning a small barrier between the client's eyes, you shine your penlight on the client's left eye.

22. You expect the left pupil to
    a. constrict.
    b. dilate.
    c. change shape.
    d. tear.

23. You expect the right pupil to _____ 1 to 3 seconds later.
    a. constrict
    b. dilate
    c. change shape
    d. exhibit nystagmus

24. This response of the left and then right pupil is an example of
    a. direct light reflex.
    b. consensual light reflex.
    c. coloboma.
    d. corneal light reflex.
    e. a and b.

25. Tears running freely from one eye of a newborn who is not crying could indicate
    a. conjunctivitis.
    b. birth trauma.
    c. imperforate lacrimal duct.
    d. exposure to an irritating substance.

CASE STUDIES

1. Frank is a 20-year-old college student who works summers for a yard service. His usual duties include mowing, edging, spraying for insects and weeds, spreading granular fertilizer, and occasional fence repair. You are seeing this client for a routine school sports physical.

   - Outline a basic and focused health history questionnaire relative to eye health for this client.

   - What especially will you focus on in regard to eye safety?

   - What particular eye assessments will you want to do relative to his exposures?

   - What specific prevention advice will you give?

   - What health promotion advice will you give?

   - Which nursing diagnoses would apply to Frank's situation?

2. Yvette is a 50-year-old secretary who has had three minor motor vehicle accidents as the driver. She admits that driving at night is stressful for her and that lights seem too bright, but also confusing and indistinct. She says that she reads at night with a book light, so as not to disturb her sleeping husband. She reports no problems at work, stating that her computer has a "nice bright screen."

   - What might you expect to discover in the health history relative to eye health?

   - What aspects of the eye assessment will be especially important for Yvette?

   - Are her complaints unusual for someone of her age? Explain.

   - What eye problems might be developing here?

CLINICAL ACTIVITIES

Assessment of the eye and vision varies considerably with age of the client, though there are absolutes that must be addressed with clients of all ages.

- Remember that the eye exam requires cooperation from the client and that parts of the exam will be fatiguing for any client. Be alert to when your client shows signs of fatigue or discomfort, and offer brief periods of rest when needed.
- Using the sample documentation form at the end of this chapter as a guideline, perform the assessment of

the eye and vision of your lab partner or willing volunteer.
- Review the advice in your text for preparation of equipment, the nurse, and the client for this assessment.

In the event that you may come in contact with body fluids, be prepared to institute appropriate precautions to protect both you and the client. Review **Appendices B and C in your text** for helpful advice.

Sample Documentation Form

Eyes and Vision

Name: _____   Date: _____

Age: _____ Gender: _____

Review of history related to the current visit:

Focused symptom analysis of current problem:

Reason for visit: _____

_____

Character: _____

Onset: _____

Duration: _____

Location: _____

Severity: _____

Associated problems: _____

Efforts to treat: _____

Current medications: _____

_____

_____

Allergies: _____

_____

History

Review of history related to eyes and vision:

YES/NO   If YES, provide details:
                                            _____

Date of last eye exam: _____

Vision

☐ ☐   Blurry vision   _____

☐ ☐   Change in vision   _____

☐ ☐   Double vision   _____

☐ ☐   Loss of vision   _____

☐ ☐   Floaters within visual field   _____

☐ ☐   Straining to see   _____

☐ ☐   Headaches related to vision   _____

☐ ☐   Glasses or contracts   _____

Eyes

☐ ☐   History of eye disease   _____

☐ ☐   Crusting or lesions on eyelids   _____

☐ ☐   Redness of eyes   _____

☐ ☐   Eye pain   _____

☐ ☐   Drainage from around eyes   _____

☐	☐	Breathing difficulties
☐	☐	Cough or cold
☐	☐	Asthma or respiratory problems
☐	☐	Allergies
☐	☐	Other

Family history of vision or eye problems:

_____

_____

Medical history relevant to eyes/vision (example: diabetes mellitus, hypertension, etc.):

_____

_____

Physical Assessment

Vision:

General evaluation of vision (glasses, contact lenses, corrective surgery):

_____

_____

Distant vision (Snellen chart or E card)

Right eye uncorrected	_____	Right eye corrected _____
Left eye uncorrected	_____	Left eye corrected _____
Both eyes uncorrected	_____	Both eyes corrected _____

Near vision (Rosenbaum or near vision card)

Right eye uncorrected	_____	Right eye corrected _____
Left eye uncorrected	_____	Left eye corrected _____
Both eyes uncorrected	_____	Both eyes corrected _____

Eyes

General characteristics—eyes (position, alignment, size):

_____

_____

Inspect and palpate.

Eyebrows (infestation, infection, shape): _____

Eyelids (opening, ptosis, tremors, redness, swelling, flaking, lashes): _____

_____

Eye orbit (lacrimal gland, lacrimal ducts, firmness, edema, pain or discomfort): _____

_____

Conjunctiva (color, discharge): _____

_____

External eyes (corneal clarity, pupil size, shape, reactivity): _____

_____

Eye muscles and movement:

Corneal light reflex: _____

Cover/uncover test: _____

Six cardinal fields of gaze: _____

Peripheral vision: _____

Opthalmoscopic Exam

	Right Eye	Left Eye
Lens clarity		
Red reflex		
Retina (color, surface characteristics)		
Disc characteristics		
Macula characteristics		

Analysis:

_____

_____

_____

Nursing diagnoses: _____

_____

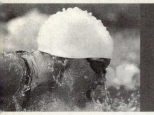

14   Ears, Nose, Mouth, and Throat

OVERVIEW

The ears, nose, mouth, and throat perform critical life functions and represent a significant portion of the body's sensory apparatus. Cranial nerves are an important part of the function of these structures, and the amount of mucous membrane involved in their structure makes them vulnerable to infection. The assessment of these structures requires both skill and knowledge on the part of the nurse.

ASSIGNMENT

CD-ROM content: Chapter 14
Companion website: www.prenhall.com/damico, Chapter 14

VOCABULARY EXERCISE

After completing the reading assignment, you should be able to define the **key terms** listed below. Refer back to the page number from main text for help.

Air conduction, 324
Auricle, 305
Bone conduction, 324
Cerumen, 306
Cochlea, 306
Eustachian tube, 306
Helix, 305
Lobule, 305
Mastoiditis, 320
Nasal polyps, 327

Ossicles, 306
Otitis externa, 315
Palate, 310
Paranasal sinuses, 307
Pinna, 305
Presbycusis, 311
Tragus, 305
Tympanic membrane, 306
Uvula, 308

ANATOMY EXERCISES

1. Label the parts of the external ear.

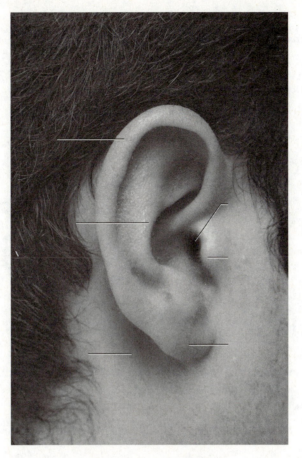

Figure 14–1 External Ear

2. What should be the consistency of the helix?

3. Label the indicated structures of the ear.

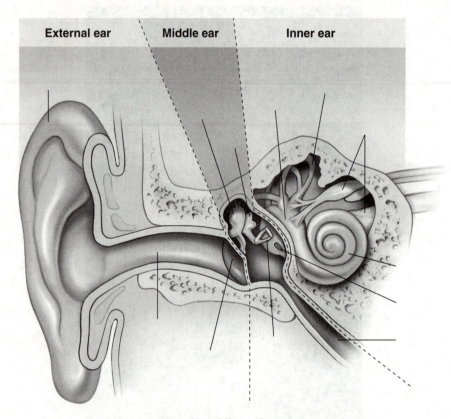

Figure 14–2 External, Middle, and Inner Ear Structures

4. What tissue lines the external auditory canal? What possible problems can occur with this tissue?

5. What portion of the eighth cranial nerve supplies the vestibule? What signs are observable to the examiner when there is dysfunction of that portion of the nerve?

6. What structures are visible on otoscopic examination?

7. Label the indicated structures of the nose, mouth, and throat.

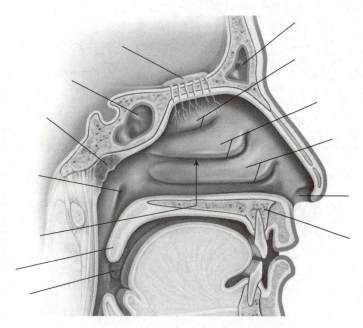

Figure 14–3 Cross Section Nose

8. How can the nurse assess the sinuses? Which of the turbinates should be visible on inspection of the internal nose?

9. Explain the importance of the eustachian tube in relation to the opening of the nasopharynx.

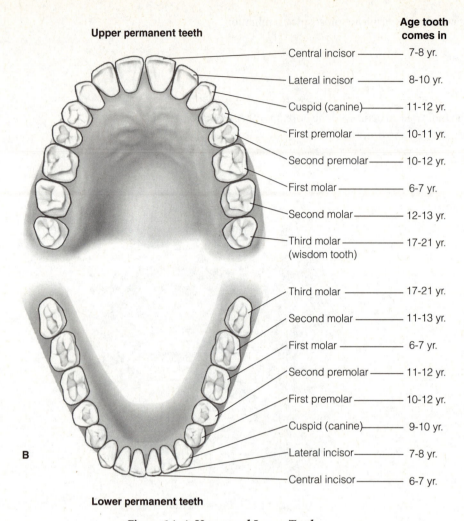

Upper permanent teeth

Tooth	Age tooth comes in
Central incisor	7-8 yr.
Lateral incisor	8-10 yr.
Cuspid (canine)	11-12 yr.
First premolar	10-11 yr.
Second premolar	10-12 yr.
First molar	6-7 yr.
Second molar	12-13 yr.
Third molar (wisdom tooth)	17-21 yr.
Third molar	17-21 yr.
Second molar	11-13 yr.
First molar	6-7 yr.
Second premolar	11-12 yr.
First premolar	10-12 yr.
Cuspid (canine)	9-10 yr.
Lateral incisor	7-8 yr.
Central incisor	6-7 yr.

B

Lower permanent teeth

Figure 14–4 Upper and Lower Teeth

10. How many teeth should be present in the adult? Look in a mirror and perform an assessment on yourself. Select one upper and one lower tooth and indicate how you would document a finding in that tooth.

STUDY FOCUS

1. If a client reports no change in hearing, why is it still important to do a hearing test?

2. What health promotion concerns relate to ear health? Does this differ in various age groups? What concerns might you have for an adolescent? For a working adult?

3. Is substance abuse a concern for the nose, mouth, sinuses, and throat? If so, why? How can you broach the subject of possible substance use without offending the client?

4. Describe what you would expect to see on otoscopic exam of the normal ear.

5. Other than actually falling down, what are some signs and symptoms of a dysfunctional vestibular system?

6. For a healthy adult, what are important health promotion questions relating to the ear, nose, mouth, and throat?

7. Under what conditions would the maxillary and frontal sinuses transilluminate? Under what conditions would they fail to transilluminate?

8. What is a more diagnostic term for swimmer's ear?

9. At what age can you expect all permanent teeth to be in place?

10. What nutritional features should be present in a diet to ensure a healthy mouth, mucous membranes, and teeth?

REVIEW QUESTIONS

1. In a unilateral conductive loss of hearing, the tone for the Weber test
  a. lateralizes to the good ear.
  b. lateralizes to the obstructed ear.
  c. does not lateralize to either ear.
  d. sounds the same in both ears.

2. In a unilateral sensorineural loss of hearing, the tone from the Weber test
  a. lateralizes to the good ear.
  b. lateralizes to the poor ear.
  c. does not lateralize to either ear.
  d. sounds the same in both ears.

3. When performing the Rinne test, which of the following would be the normal response?
  a. BC > AC 1:2
  b. AC = BC 2:1
  c. AC > BC 2:1
  d. none of the above

4. Proper direction of the otoscope along the ear canal is of great importance to client comfort because the canal is lined with a friable mucous membrane.
  a. true
  b. false

5. Increased amounts of cerumen in an ear canal can cause _____ hearing loss.
  a. conductive
  b. temporary
  c. sensorineural
  d. indiscernible

6. Drainage from the ear canal can include
  a. cerumen.
  b. blood.
  c. purulent debris.
  d. cerebral spinal fluid.
  e. all of the above.

7. Pain on manipulation of the external ear may indicate
  a. perichondritis (inflammation of cartilage).
  b. otitis externa (swimmer's ear).
  c. foreign object in the canal.
  d. all of the above.

Matching: Match the descriptive diagnostic term with the choices listed after question 10.

8. infection of the middle ear _____

9. infection of the canal _____

10. fluid behind the tympanic membrane _____
  a. otitis externa
  b. otitis media
  c. serous otitis

Mark "a" for true and "b" for false. External inspection of the ear may detect:

11. malignancy _____

12. infection/inflammation _____

13. possibility of renal defects _____

14. congenital defects _____

15. subtle hearing loss _____

16. Lips and buccal mucosa should be evaluated for
  a. skin lesions.
  b. color and muscle tone.
  c. infectious processes.
  d. allergic signs.
  e. all of the above.

17. Examination of the tongue may reveal
  a. nutritional deficiencies.
  b. neurologic pathology.
  c. immune dysfunction.
  d. all of the above.

18. Presence of mucous discharge on the posterior pharynx always indicates infection of the pharynx.
  a. true
  b. false

19. The sinuses evaluated by inspection, palpation, and percussion are
    a. sphenoid and ethmoid.
    b. frontal and maxillary.
    c. splanchnic.
    d. a and b.

20. Examination of the mouth should be done
    a. with dentures in place.
    b. with dentures removed.
    c. a and b.

21. The teeth are assessed for
    a. color, placement, and caries.
    b. presence, shape, position, looseness, and caries.
    c. absence, position, and color.
    d. symmetry, color, and lesions.

22. Tonsils are inspected for
    a. presence.
    b. size.
    c. crypts.
    d. exudates.
    e. all of the above.

23. Oral mucosa should be examined for
    a. color and texture.
    b. masses.
    c. leukoplakia.
    d. friability (bleeds easily).
    e. all of the above.

24. Epistaxis is a deviation of the nasal septum.
    a. true
    b. false

25. The presence of swollen, boggy, pale, and gray nasal mucosa may indicate
    a. chronic allergy.
    b. chronic infection.
    c. nasal polyps.
    d. cocaine abuse.

CASE STUDIES

1. Carolyn, age 30, presents complaining of a sore throat. She says this is the third one this year but all have occurred in the last 2 months. No one else in the family has had sore throats during this time. Carolyn has no chronic health problems, and her vital signs are within normal limits.

   • What focused interview would you plan to take from Carolyn?

   • What physical assessments have already been done?

   • What physical assessment would you do now?

   • What nursing diagnoses could apply to Carolyn's complaints?

2. Armondo Beliz, age 43, has been smoking since he was 9 years old. Advised to give that up 3 years ago, he has been using chewing tobacco ever since. He reports having diminished taste sensation and some "numb" spots in his mouth.

   • What additional health history (family, past medical, current) do you need?

   • In review of systems, on which systems will you focus?

   • What specific physical assessments should be performed now?

- What physical findings would you look for specifically in the mouth? In the nose? In the throat?

- What health promotion strategies would you recommend?

CLINICAL ACTIVITIES

Be sure that the clinical area is quiet when doing a hearing evaluation so that results are based on true hearing ability and not contaminated by background noise.

▶ Using sample documentation form at the end of the chapter as a guideline, pursue any findings with additional questions or assessment findings.

Clients complaining of nose, mouth, and throat problems may be a danger to the nurse even for history taking.

▶ Be sure to protect with self hygiene, gloves for the assessment, and goggles if the client is coughing or sneezing.

▶ Review **Appendices B and C in your text** for specific information on protection of the nurse and client.

▶ Perform a complete ear, nose, mouth, and throat history and physical assessment on your lab partner or willing volunteer.

▶ Following the assessment, even for the well client, correctly dispose of or clean all equipment.

Sample Documentation Form

Ears, Nose, Mouth, and Throat

Name: _____ Date: _____

Age: _____ Gender: _____

History

Review of history related to nose, mouth, throat, and ears:
_____

YES/NO   If YES, provide details:
_____

Nose

☐ ☐ Problem with your nose _____
☐ ☐ Trauma/surgery to nose _____
☐ ☐ Problem with your sinuses _____
☐ ☐ Allergies (ask about presentation) _____
☐ ☐ Injury of or surgery on nose _____
☐ ☐ Change in smell ability _____
☐ ☐ Nasal obstruction _____
☐ ☐ Cold and/or sneezing _____
☐ ☐ Snorting or sniffing substances _____
☐ ☐ Snoring _____
☐ ☐ Nosebleeds _____
☐ ☐ Sinus infection _____
☐ ☐ Use of nasal sprays _____
                          Type spray: _____
                          Length of use: _____

Mouth

☐ ☐ Problem with your mouth _____
☐ ☐ Lesions or sores in mouth _____
☐ ☐ Swollen or bleeding gums _____
☐ ☐ Problem with your teeth _____
☐ ☐ Difficulty chewing _____
☐ ☐ Lost teeth _____
☐ ☐ Wear dentures (fit) _____
☐ ☐ Last dental checkup Date: _____
☐ ☐ Change in taste _____
☐ ☐ Sensitivity to cold or hot _____
☐ ☐ Bad breath _____
☐ ☐ Painful tongue _____
☐ ☐ Tongue, mouth, lip piercing _____

Throat

☐ ☐ Hoarseness _____
☐ ☐ Loss of voice _____
☐ ☐ Difficulty Swallowing _____
☐ ☐ Frequent sore throats _____
☐ ☐ Frequent infections _____

Tobacco Products

☐ ☐ Smoke cigarettes _____

☐ ☐ Smoke pipe _____

☐ ☐ Chew tobacco _____

☐ ☐ Related problems _____

Ears and Hearing

☐ ☐ Ear disease or trauma _____

☐ ☐ Tinnitus _____

☐ ☐ Dizziness or vertigo _____

☐ ☐ Medications _____

☐ ☐ Occupational noise exposure _____

☐ ☐ Discharge from ears _____

☐ ☐ Infections _____

☐ ☐ Otalgia _____

☐ ☐ Allergies _____

☐ ☐ Hearing problems _____

    If Yes: One or both ears

                Best sounds heard _____

                Difficult sounds _____

                How managed

☐ ☐ Hearing aid use _____

Current medications: _____

_____

Family history of nose, mouth, throat, ears, or hearing problems: _____

_____

Allergies: _____

_____

Health promotion/specific prevention behaviors related to mouth, nose, throat, ears, or hearing:

_____

_____

Current Problem

  Focused analysis of current problem:

      Character: _____

      Onset: _____

      Duration: _____

      Location: _____

      Severity: _____

      Association problems: _____

      Efforts to treat: _____

Physical Assessment

Inspect and palpate.

Nose:

Appearance (symmetry, placement, lesions, scars): _____
_____

Nasal discharge (amount, characteristics, odor): _____
_____

Nasal patency (air movement, bilateral patency, septum position and character): _____
_____

Olfactory nerve (Cranial nerve I—smell, test bilaterally): _____

Sinus tenderness (inspect and palpate sinuses): _____
_____

Mouth:

General characteristics (hygiene, teeth, lips, smile, ease of movement): _____
_____

Teeth (number, repair, alignment, hygiene, placement/stability, tenderness): _____
_____

Gums (lesions, color, bleeding, swelling): _____

Hard and soft palate (color, pigmentation, moisture, lesions): _____
_____

Mucous membrane (color, pigmentation, moisture, salivary glands): _____
_____

Tongue (color, position, exudate, lumps, masses): _____
_____

Throat:

General characteristics (swallowing, lesions): _____
_____

Posterior pharynx (color, swelling, exudate, tonsils, tonsillar pillar, uvula): _____
_____

Glossopharyngeal and vagus nerves (cranial nerves IX and X; movement of uvula, soft palate, and gag reflex): _____

Ears and Hearing:

Inspect and palpate.

Skin of ears (color, tone, and texture): _____

Auricles (position and shape, lesions): _____

Auditory meatus (patency, drainage): _____

Ear alignment with eyes: _____

Pinna, tragus (characteristics, position): _____

Mastoid process: _____

Drainage, inflammation, tenderness, lesions: _____

Otoscopic examination:

Ear canal (color, characteristics, cerumen, lesions, foreign objects, drainage): _____

_____

Tympanic membrane (color, intactness, landmarks, characteristics): _____

_____

Hearing acuity:

Watch or whisper (sound characteristics): ☐ Expected

Describe: _____

Rinne test (air conduction > bone conduction): ☐ Expected

Describe: _____

Weber test (sound lateralization): ☐ Expected

Describe: _____

Vestibular assessment:

Romberg test (balance maintained): ☐ Yes   ☐ No

Describe: _____

Analysis:

_____

_____

Nursing diagnoses: _____

_____

Respiratory System 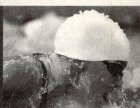 15

OVERVIEW

This chapter will help you recall the structure, function, and techniques to be used for the assessment of the respiratory system. The **anatomy** of the chest and lungs is critical to its function and is the first point of assessment. The shape of the chest and its ability to expand and contract determine ventilation. The purpose of the system, along with the cardiovascular system, is to provide life-giving oxygen and remove gaseous by-products of metabolism. All systems affect one another as you have already learned, though it's tempting to see the impact of

the respiratory system as of exceptional importance to all systems. Think about the impact of a respiratory malfunction on the cardiovascular and neurologic systems, as well as skin, musculoskeletal, gastrointestinal, and reproductive systems.

At the completion of this chapter and its activities, you will be able to assess chest shape, size, and movement; identify expected and adventitious lung sounds; and evaluate voice sounds auscultated on the chest.

ASSIGNMENT

CD-ROM content: Chapter 15
Companion website: www.prenhall.com/damico, Chapter 15, especially Toolbox

VOCABULARY EXERCISE

After completing the reading assignment, you should be able to define the **key terms** listed below. Refer back to the page number from the main text for help.

Adventitious sounds, 378
Angle of Louis, 353
Bronchial sounds, 377
Bronchophony, 379
Bronchovesicular sounds, 377
Dullness, 375
Dyspnea, 353
Egophony, 379
Eupnea, 353
Fremitus, 373

Landmarks, 353
Manubrium, 353
Mediastinum, 349
Resonance, 374
Respiratory cycle, 349
Rhonchi, 378
Tracheal sounds, 377
Vesicular sounds, 377
Wheezes, 378
Whispered pectoriloquy, 379

ANATOMY EXERCISES

1. Label each body part using the line provided.

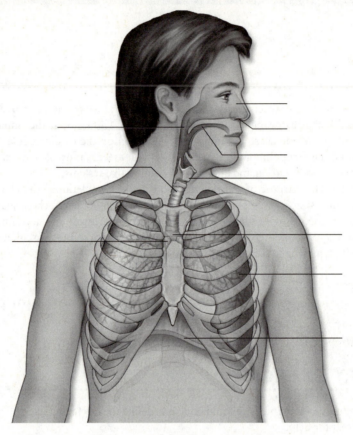

Figure 15–1

2. Note the entirety of the respiratory system (from nose to alveoli). What impact could sinus or oral infections have on the lower tract?

3. Judging by the contour of the right and left bronchus, in which might a foreign object more easily lodge?

4. Label each bony landmark.

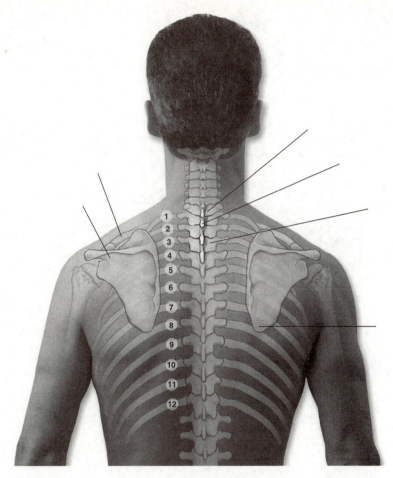

Figure 15–2

5. Note that the respiratory system begins at the mouth and nares. Of what clinical significance is this?

6. Label landmarks.

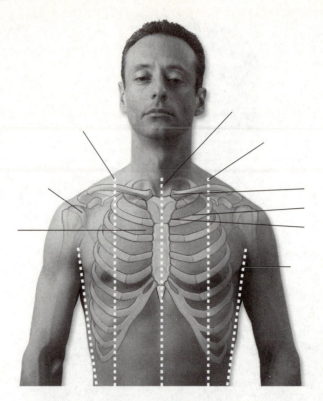

Figure 15–3

7. Label landmarks.

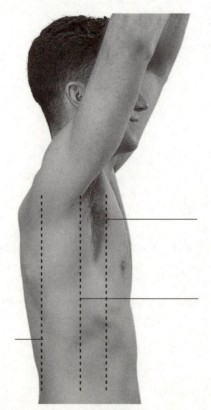

Figure 15–4

8. Indicate the type of breath sound expected in each location.

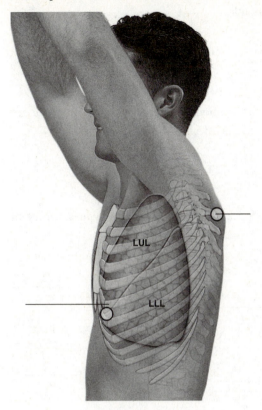

Figure 15–5

9. Indicate which normal breath sounds could be auscultated in each area.

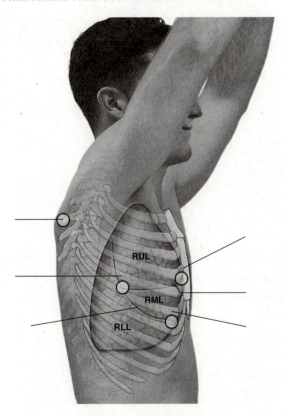

Figure 15–6

10. On Figures 15–5 and 15–6 label those areas where you would expect to hear tracheal or bronchial sounds, and bronchovesicular or vesicular sounds.

11. If you were to hear the following adventitious sounds: rales/crackles, rhonchi, and wheezes, where would they most likely be located?

12. Select and label the following: eupnea, sighing, bradypnea tachypnea, hyperventilation, hypoventilation, Cheyne-Stokes, Biots.

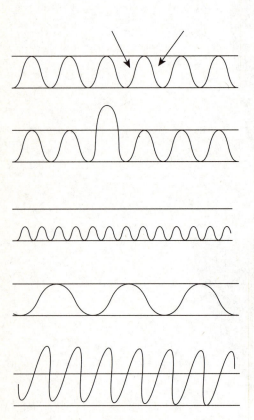

Figure 15–7

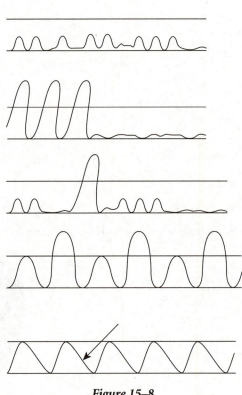

Figure 15–8

STUDY FOCUS

1. List questions related to the respiratory system that will reveal a client's lifestyle.

2. How would a history of substance abuse relate to the respiratory system?

3. What physiological function do the trachea and bronchus perform? What would be some concerns if that tissue should become infected?

4. What is the significance of limited respiratory excursion? How would you determine if excursion was physiological?

5. What conditions are associated with absent breath sounds over a specific lung area?

6. How soon could advanced findings such as stridor or intercostal retractions be observed in a client complaining of respiratory illness?

7. Of what clinical use is the angle of Louis?

REVIEW QUESTIONS

1. The purpose of the side-to-side pattern used during respiratory assessment in percussion and in auscultation is to
   a. prevent fatiguing the client.
   b. tightly organize the assessment.
   c. allow comparison of like areas of lung tissue.
   d. conserve time.

2. Soft, fine breath sounds can be auscultated
   a. immediately above the clavicles.
   b. in all of the axillary lines.
   c. immediately above the diaphragm; anterior.
   d. immediately above the diaphragm; posterior.
   e. in all of the above areas.

3. Thoracic expansion assesses which of the following characteristics?
   a. vibrations
   b. voice sounds
   c. breath sounds
   d. chest movement

4. You are percussing your client's posterior chest at $T_{10} \rightarrow T_{12}$ space, midscapular line, and obtain a flat percussion note. *Most likely* you are percussing over
   a. normal lung.
   b. diaphragm.
   c. trachea.
   d. tumor.
   e. barrel chest.

5. To inspect the chest, you should observe
   a. while the client holds breath.
   b. while the client breathes naturally.
   c. with your palm on the client's chest.
   d. after the client begins to cough.

6. Percussion of the back should be done with the client's arms folded in front, to
   a. prevent attacks of coughing.
   b. make the scapulae protrude.
   c. distinguish thudlike from drumlike sounds.
   d. expose maximum lung area.

7. The diaphragm of the stethoscope is better than the bell for auscultation of the lungs because it
   a. filters extraneous sounds.
   b. amplifies all types of sound.
   c. best transmits high-pitched sounds.
   d. pinpoints focal sound areas.
   e. fits flat against the chest.

8. In the case of consolidated lung or solid tumor, tactile fremitus would be
   a. increased.
   b. decreased.

Matching:

9. predictable difficulty breathing while reclining _____

10. unexpected or "added" finding _____

11. difficult or painful breathing _____

12. respiratory rate greater than 20 (adult) _____
    a. tachypnea
    b. orthopnea
    c. adventitious
    d. hyperventilation
    e. dyspnea

13. Crepitus and friction rubs are adventitious sounds discovered *only* on respiratory auscultation.
    a. true
    b. false

14. Crackles are
    a. caused by air passing through moisture.
    b. heard most often during inspiration.
    c. found in lung bases with congestive heart failure.
    d. all of the above.

Matching:

15. physiological sound heard at lung apices _____

16. dry rubbing or grating sound on auscultation _____

17. physiological sound heard at lung bases _____

18. continuous high-pitched almost musical sound _____
    a. rales/crackles
    b. wheezes
    c. pleural friction rub
    d. vesicular breath sounds
    e. bronchovesicular sounds

19. When auscultating the lungs, listen to the breath sounds
    a. during expiration.
    b. during inspiration.
    c. for 30 seconds.
    d. throughout inspiration and expiration.

20. Stridor, wheezes, and grunts describe _____ of respiration.
    a. quality
    b. rate
    c. pattern

21. In the physiological thorax, stethoscopic ausculation of voice sounds reveals
    a. egophony.
    b. clear, distinct voice sounds.
    c. loudest sounds at the periphery.
    d. muffled, indistinct voice sounds.

CASE STUDIES

1. A 16-year-old girl presents in the school nurse's office seeking advice regarding a persistent cough. The girl is well nourished, has a good attendance record at school, and is on grade with her studies.

   • What health history information do you need?

- What physical assessment techniques will you use?

- What etiologies for a cough come to your mind? How would you rule any of these in or out in thinking of a possible diagnosis?

2. You are assigned a client in your clinical rotation in an acute care setting who is diagnosed with pneumonia. What will you expect to see when you meet this client?

- The general survey may reveal what observations? For example, posture, skin color, facial expression, and so on.

- What changes would you expect in vital signs? List each and give likely changes.

- What would the nursing diagnoses associated with this medical diagnosis be?

CLINICAL ACTIVITIES

Using the two sample documentation forms at the end of the chapter as a guideline, perform these activities with your lab partner or, if possible, a client in your clinical assignment. Be very cautious with respiratory clients so that you are protected from contamination with droplets and/or any body fluids. Review **Appendices B and C in your text** for helpful guidelines for your protection.

HISTORY TAKING AND DOCUMENTATION
Preparation

1. List areas of relevance to the respiratory system that would be family history for a client.
2. Identify health history questions that support health promotion activities used by the client. Think about lifestyle choices and also environmental factors.
3. List past medical history that would be specific to the respiratory system.
4. List complaints that would be specific to the respiratory system.

Physical Assessment

1. Assess respirations. What aspects of breathing can be assessed without special tools? Evaluate rate, rhythm, quality, effort, and pattern. Observe the client's skin color, posture, apparent energy, manifestations of pain, and shape of the fingernails. What are the expected findings for the listed parameters? Document your actual findings.
2. Assess chest symmetry and movement. Evaluate chest shape, movement on expansion, and symmetry of chest. What are expected findings for shape? What techniques can be used to determine shape? What is a minimum amount of chest expansion for the healthy adult? Document your actual findings. What disease conditions are associated with problems of poor chest movement? What diseases cause changes in chest shape?
3. Evaluate breath sounds. Using the diaphragm of the stethoscope, auscultate the client's chest. What type of breath sounds should you hear in the area immediately surrounding the sternum anteriorly and the vertebral column posteriorly? Which breath sounds do you expect to hear above the clavicles? Which do you expect to hear in the axillary regions, and which in the areas just above the diaphragm? How would you document your findings? Which three aspects of assessment of breath sounds should always be documented?
4. Find a discussion of asthma in your textbook. What are the historical factors that would point toward this disease? Would there likely be family history? What past medical history might be expected? What other coexisting diseases could be present?
5. If your client complained of coughing, what would you need to know about the cough? Take a full history of a cough.

Sample Documentation Form

Respiratory Assessment

Client name _____ Age _____ Sex _____ Occupation _____

Provider _____

General Health History (relative to respiratory)

Family history _____

Past medical history _____

Focused Health History

Client complaint _____

Symptom	No	Yes, Explain
Cough		
Chest pain		
Dyspnea		
Exposures		
Other		

Physical Assessment

General Survey

1. Attitude/posture_____
2. Skin color _____
3. Alertness _____
4. Vital signs _____

Inspection

1. Respiratory rate, rhythm, quality _____
2. Respiratory effort, use of accessory muscles _____
3. Thorax: shape, movement (anterior, posterior, lateral) _____

Palpation

1. Symmetrical chest expansion _____
2. Masses, points of tenderness_____
3. Tactile fremitus _____
4. Trachea position _____

Percussion

1. Percussion note and location over lung _____
2. Diaphragmatic excursion _____

Auscultation (indicate tracheal/bronchial, bronchovesicular, vesicular, and location)

1. Anterior _____
2. Lateral, right and left _____
3. Posterior _____

4. Adventitious breath sounds (type and location) _____

5. Voice sounds _____

6. Adventitious voice sounds and location _____

Assessment/Analysis

_____

_____

Nursing Diagnosis

_____

Alternate Documentation Form

RESPIRATORY SYSTEM

Name: _____ Date: _____

Age: _____ Gender: _____

History

Review of the respiratory system: _____

YES/NO   If YES, provide details:

☐	☐	Allergies	_____
☐	☐	Fever	_____
☐	☐	Asthma, wheezing	_____
☐	☐	Tobacco use	_____
☐	☐	Medications	_____
☐	☐	Cough	_____
☐	☐	Sputum production	_____
☐	☐	Hemoptysis	_____
☐	☐	Chest pain	_____
☐	☐	Shortness of breath	_____
☐	☐	Occupational risk factors	_____
☐	☐	Environmental risk factors	_____
☐	☐	Respiratory disease history	_____
☐	☐	Use of aerosols or inhalants	_____
☐	☐	Cardiac history	_____
☐	☐	Chest trauma	_____

Social history (occupational and home exposures, fitness activies, safety habits [seat belts, etc.]):

_____

_____

_____

_____

Family history related to respiratory system:

_____

_____

_____

_____

Focused symptom analysis of current problem:

Problem statement: _____

    Characteristics: _____

    Onset: _____

    Duration: _____

    Location: _____

    Severity: _____

    Associated problems: _____

    Efforts to treat: _____

Physical Assessment

  Vital Signs

    Temperature: _____   Pulse: _____

    Respirations (rate, rhythm, quality): _____

    Blood pressure: _____

  Inspection

    Skin (color, tone, texture): _____

    Thorax (shape, symmetry, movement, use of accessory muscles): _____

    Breathing (rate, pattern, audible sounds): _____

    Posture: _____

    Alertness: _____

    Nails (oxygenation, clubbing): _____

  Palpation

    Skin (temperature, tenderness, unusual sensations): _____

    Trachea (position, mobility): _____

    Thoracic excursion (symmetry, anterior/posterior): _____

    Tactile fremitus (characteristics): _____

    Ribs and thorax (shape, symmetry, tenderness, masses): _____

    Respiratory excursion (findings): _____

  Percussion

  Tones over thorax (describe tones and location):

    Describe: _____

    Anterior: _____

    Posterior: _____

Auscultation

Breath sounds (apices, anterior lungs, posterior lungs, lateral lung fields—anterior/posterior):
Respiratory sounds in each location:

Describe: _____

Anterior: _____

Posterior: _____

_____

Adventitious sounds (if present, describe): _____

_____

_____

Vocal resonance (sound characteristics): _____

Analysis:

_____

_____

_____

Nursing diagnoses: _____

_____

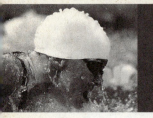

16 Breasts and Axillae

OVERVIEW

Breast health, as with any body part, is integral to the whole body. Vulnerability to cancer, however, makes assessment of the breast of even greater importance. At our current level of knowledge, early discovery of breast cancer is the only tool we have in defense. A thorough clinical assessment and excellent client teaching for breast self-exam are lifesaving skills that nurses can develop to offer their clients.

ASSIGNMENT

CD-ROM content: Chapter 16
Companion website: www.prenhall.com/damico, Chapter 16

VOCABULARY EXERCISE

After completing the reading assignment, you should be able to define the **key terms** listed below. Refer back to the page number from the main text for help.

Acini cells, 398
Areola, 398
Colostrum, 402
Galactorrhea, 415
Gynecomastia, 402

Mammary ridge, 399
Montgomery's glands, 398
Peau d'orange, 409
Suspensory ligaments, 398

ANATOMY EXERCISES

1. Label the anatomical structures of the breast.

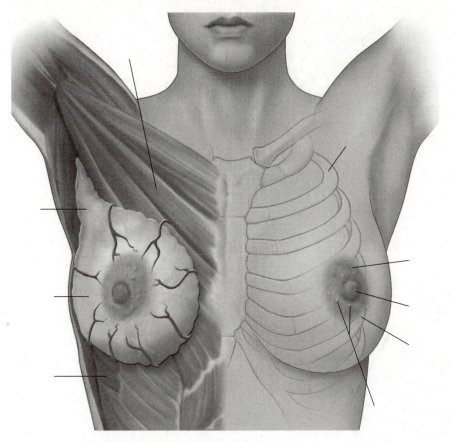

Figure 16–1

2. Note the extension of the breast up toward the axillae called the tail of Spence. Plan to continue the breast assessment through this tissue. Note, and teach your client to note, the contour of the breast when the arms are raised as in this drawing. All should be symmetrical.

3. What pattern of assessment is recommended for a comprehensive breast exam?

4. What other positions for the client make up a thorough breast exam?

5. Label the lymph structures of the breast.

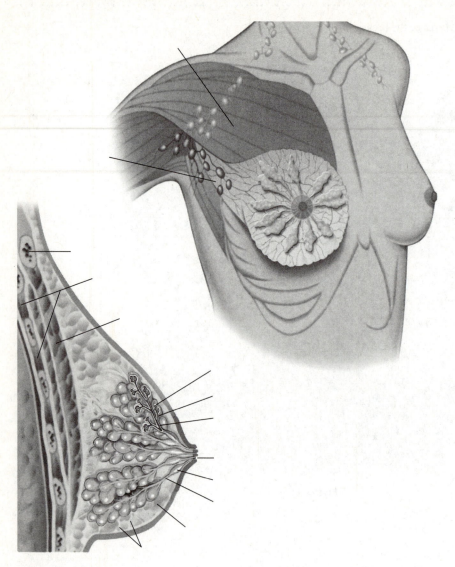

Figure 16–2

6. Note the different types of tissue in the breast. Do you think this makes assessment easier or more difficult?

7. How would you explain to a woman the variations of tissue in her breast?

8. How does a woman's breast tissue change over time, in days?

9. How does her breast change over time, in years? How does this change assessment?

10. What significant factor is different between the male and the female breast for assessment?

11. Label indicated lymph nodes.

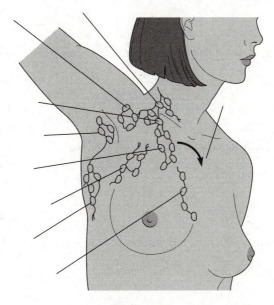

Figure 16–3

12. Assessment of regional lymph nodes is an integral part of breast assessment. What would be the significance of a swollen lymph node?

13. One small cluster of lymph nodes associated with the breast is not shown here. What is it?

STUDY FOCUS

1. What basic historical information must the nurse have in order to draw any conclusions regarding the condition of the breasts? (Give at least three.) Why is LMP (last menstrual period) of great importance?

2. Family history is very important to evaluation of risk. What degree of relative having breast cancer is of most concern?

3. Examination of the skin of the breast is relative to cancer in two ways. Identify these potential risks.

4. What are the five positions in which the breasts should be examined?

5. What is the purpose of assessment in five various positions?

6. How does skin texture relate to breast cancer assessment?

7. How does exam of the male breast differ from that of the female?

8. When would you recommend a female client perform self breast examination (BSE)?

REVIEW QUESTIONS

1. An enlargement or swelling of a lymph node can indicate
   a. infection in a region drained by the node.
   b. a malignancy in the lymph region.
   c. allergic responses.
   d. infiltration by foreign substances.
   e. all/any of the above.

2. BSE is best accomplished by women with menstrual cycles at the time of
   a. ovulation.
   b. menstrual bleeding.
   c. 10 days prior to menstrual bleeding.
   d. 5 to 8 days following day one of menstrual bleeding.

3. Your advice to men, regarding BSE, is
   a. do not be concerned; male breast carcinoma rates are very low.
   b. have a mammogram with your exam.
   c. perform a BSE monthly.
   d. check your breast tissue once a year.

4. The most effective intervention against breast cancer is
   a. prevention.
   b. early detection.
   c. rigorous chemotherapy.
   d. health promotion activities.

5. Following are ominous signs of breast disease found on history and/or physical exam:
   a. unequal size breast (i.e., right breast larger than left breast), inverted nipples
   b. skin texture that is rougher or dimpled as compared to surrounding skin
   c. drainage from a nipple not associated with lactation or stimulation
   d. a small nodule fixed to underlying tissue
   e. b, c, and d

6. Swollen mammary nodes associated with the presence of a nodule in the breast tissue
   a. are always associated with malignancy.
   b. give cause for relief (not usually associated with malignancy).
   c. should be aggressively evaluated.

7. The clock face pattern of breast assessment by palpation discussed in your text
   a. is the only pattern capable of thorough assessment of breast tissue.
   b. is a convention used to offer consistency in teaching BSE techniques.
   c. is inferior to the mammogram.
   d. should be used only with young, small-breasted women.

8. Your client complains of tenderness generally throughout her breasts as you palpate her breast tissue. Important data relevant to this finding include
   a. her usual tolerance of pain.
   b. relationship of exam date to her menstrual cycle.
   c. her gravida.
   d. her age.
   e. your experience as an examiner.

9. Your best recommendations specific to *breast* health protection to a 28-year-old female concerned about breast cancer would include
   a. diet and exercise standards.
   b. caution related to specific environmental exposures.
   c. monthly BSE and yearly exam by provider.
   d. mammogram.
   e. genetic testing.

10. Regarding the recent controversy about hormone replacement therapy (HRT), the following is now generally accepted to be true:
    a. Postmenopausal hormone replacement therapy is associated with some small degree of increase in breast cancer.
    b. Women should not hesitate to use HRT.
    c. HRT offers protection against cardiovascular disease.
    d. HRT may offer some protection against dementia.

11. Persistent eczematous dermatitis of the nipples and surrounding tissues, absent these symptoms on any other area of the body,
    a. is suggestive of poor hygiene.
    b. may be associated with a malignant process.
    c. is likely fibrocystic breast disease.

12. Breasts of unequal size usually indicate _____.

13. Differences between fat breasts and gynecomastia, discernible on physical exam, include
    a. size.
    b. texture of tissue.
    c. symmetry of nipple.
    d. color of skin.

14. A lymphatic exam should always accompany the breast exam. Lymph tissue usually associated with a breast exam include (circle all that apply)
    a. axillary.
    b. epitrochlear.
    c. mediastinal.
    d. inguinal.
    e. supraclavicular.

15. Fibroadenomas are
    a. precancerous tumors.
    b. complications of selected medications.
    c. common in postmenopausal women.
    d. benign tumors most common in ages teens to early 20s.

CASE STUDIES

1. Angie is a 28-year-old female who is planning to get pregnant in the next year. She would very much like to breast-feed but has serious and upsetting doubts that this may not be possible. She reports that she has had fibrocystic breast disease since her late teens. She was told that this is a benign condition, but she worries that her breast tissue has been damaged and that she will not be able to breastfeed her baby.

   - What history would you need from Angie relative to breast health? Family history, past medical history, and present state of breast health?

   - What physical assessment would you plan to do?

   - What can you tell Angie about fibrocystic breast disease?

   - What relationship might Angie's fibrocystic breast disease have to her ability to breastfeed?

   - What nursing diagnoses might apply to Angie at this stage of assessment?

2. Cheryl, 57 years old, reports that it has been 4 years since her last menstrual period. During her annual examination, she is surprised to hear you say that she should be doing a breast exam every month. "I thought that was all over when I quit menstruating!" she says.

   - What will you tell Cheryl about her risk of breast cancer and the need for continued BSE?

   - What historical information do you need from your client?

   - What specifically will you do relative to her breast health during the physical exam?

   - What can you tell Cheryl about the consistency of breast tissue after menopause as compared to her earlier years?

   - What nursing diagnosis applies to Cheryl?

CLINICAL ACTIVITIES

After reading Chapter 16 carefully, critique your own efforts at BSE.

▶ Identify your risk factors by reflecting on your past medical history and your family history of cancer in general and breast cancer specifically.

▶ Do your breast exam standing in front of a mirror, and then in the supine position.

▶ Has your reading changed your BSE method? If so, in what way? What thoughts and feelings come to mind as you do your exam? Will this experience assist you in being more empathetic with your client?

Now you are ready to perform a clinical breast exam on your partner or on models provided by your nursing instructor.

▶ Be sure to provide your client with maximum privacy, having appropriate draping and support available.

▶ When working with a client or with a willing volunteer, this is an opportune time to teach techniques of breast self-exam and to suggest a routine for making this a part of the client's self-care (for example, 3 days after her menses or when she pays a monthly bill).

▶ Use the sample documentation form at the end of the chapter as a guideline. Document history and physical assessment.

Wear gloves if there is any possibility of coming into contact with body fluids such as a discharge from the nipples. Gloves reduce sensation somewhat for the examining hand, but the protection of the nurse should never be compromised. Explain to the client that you do this for his or her protection. Review Standard Precautions in Appendices B and C in your text.

Sample Documentation Form

Breast and Lymphatics

Name: _____ Date: _____

Age: _____ Gender: _____

History

Review of history related to the breasts and lymphatic system:

YES/NO	If YES, provide details:

Past Medical History

☐	☐	Breast disease	_____
☐	☐	Cancer history	_____
☐	☐	Pregnancies	_____
☐	☐	Breastfeeding	_____
☐	☐	Hormonal medications	_____
☐	☐	Lymph node enlargement	_____
☐	☐	Lymph node pain	_____
☐	☐	Breast lump(s)	_____
☐	☐	Nipple changes/discharge	_____
☐	☐	Rash or skin changes (breast)	_____
☐	☐	Breast self-exam (BSE)	_____
☐	☐	Surgery, biopsy	_____

If Yes Date: _____ Details: _____

Family History

☐	☐	Breast cancer	_____
☐	☐	Other breast diseases	_____
☐	☐	Cancer history	_____

Review of history related to the current visit

☐	☐	Breast discomfort	_____
☐	☐	Breast mass, thickening, lump(s)	_____
☐	☐	Nipple discharge	_____
☐	☐	Breast problems during menses	_____
☐	☐	Lymph node discomfort	_____
☐	☐	Perform breast self-exam	_____
☐	☐	Examination by Health care provider	_____

Focused symptom analysis of current problem:

Reason for visit: _____

_____

Character: _____

Onset: _____

Duration: _____

Location: _____

Severity: _____

Associated problems: _____

Efforts to treat: _____

Current medications: _____

_____

_____

Allergies: _____

_____

Last Mammogram

Date: _____

Results: _____

Physical Assessment

Inspect and palpate the breasts with client sitting and lying.

Inspection:

Size and symmetry of breasts: _____

Skin color and texture (discoloration, retractions, dimpling, lumps): _____

_____

Nipple placement, color texture, characteristics (discoloration, dimpling, discharge, lesions, cracking): _____

Axilla (skin, swelling, redness, lesions): _____

Palpation

Breasts (tissue characteristics, lumps, masses, thickness, tenderness, pain, dimpling): _____

_____

Nipples (discharge, pain, lesions, characteristics): _____

_____

Lymph (size, shape, consistency, node enlargement, firmness, redness, matting, pain, tenderness):

_____

Axilla and nodes (size, shape, consistency, mobility, matting, enlargement, tenderness):

_____

_____

Breast self-exam:

Knowledge? _____

Performance? _____

Teaching required? _____

Analysis:

_____

_____

_____

_____

Nursing diagnoses: _____

_____

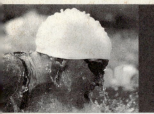

17 Cardiovascular System

OVERVIEW

We've known for some time that cardiovascular disease is America's number-one cause of death. Sadly, women are now well represented as equal victims of these illnesses. Now we are told that we are dying and being made ill by our very lifestyle. This is bad news but also good news for nurses. Although we can't do much about genetics, we can do a lot to identify lifestyle risks and we can teach about healthy lifestyle modifications. All begins with, and depends upon, a thorough assessment.

ASSIGNMENT

CD-ROM content: Chapter 17, especially heart sounds
Companion website: www.prenhall.com/damico, Chapter 17, especially Toolbox

VOCABULARY EXERCISE

After completing the reading assignment, you should be able to define the **key terms** listed below. Refer back to the page number from the main text for help.

Atrioventricular node (AV node), 434
Atrioventricular valves, 429
Bruit, 461
Bundle branches, 436
Bundle of His, 434
Cardiac conduction system, 434
Cardiac cycle, 437
Cardiac output, 439
Diastole, 429
Electrocardiogram, 438
Endocardium, 428
Epicardium, 427
Heart, 426
Heart murmur, 431
Infective endocarditis, 455
Left atrium, 428
Left ventricle, 428

Marfan's syndrome, 453
Mediastinal space, 426
Myocardium, 428
Pericardium, 426
Purkinje fibers, 436
Right atrium, 428
Right ventricle, 428
S_1, 429
S_2, 429
Semilunar valves, 429
Sinoatrial node (SA node), 434
Sternum, 437
Stroke volume, 439
Systole, 429
Thrill, 458
Visceral layer of pericardium, 426
Xanthelasma, 453

ANATOMY EXERCISES

1. Label all lines indicating auscultatory areas and bony landmarks for assessment of heart sounds.

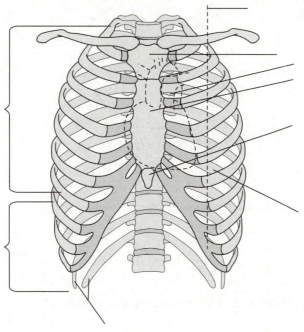

Figure 17–1

2. When will you use the bell and when will you use the diaphragm of your stethoscope in cardiac auscultation?

3. Are all unexpected sounds best heard with the bell?

4. Where on the chest would S_1 be best heard? Where would S_2 be best heard?

5. Why would the individual heart sounds be heard differently at different anatomical locations?

6. Label the cardiac cycle. Label the boxes with the heart sound that would occur in that phase of the cardiac cycle.

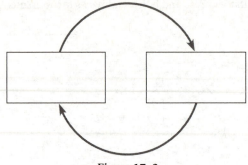

Figure 17–2

7. How does the nurse use the cardiac cycle to assess unexpected sounds?

8. What factors should be documented when an unexpected sound is detected?

9. Label all lines indicating components of the heart.

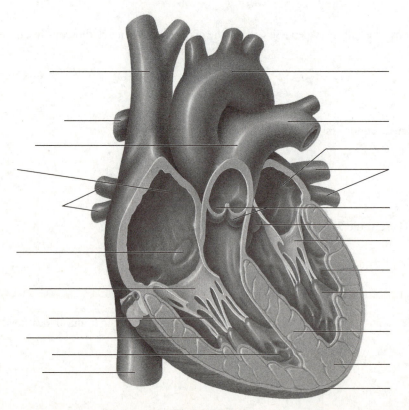

Figure 17–3

10. Once labeled, trace the path of blood flow through the heart with a colored marker.

11. Note the difference in muscle wall thickness between auricles and ventricles. Why is this the case?

STUDY FOCUS

1. Why is stress of such great importance to the cardiovascular system? What are the actual physiological factors involved?

2. Why do you suppose that African Americans have an increased rate of coronary heart disease? What implications does this have for potential nursing interventions?

3. What are the factors in the head and neck physical exam that reveal cardiac risk factors?

4. What chronic diseases have negative effects on the cardiovascular system?

5. What acute diseases have negative effects on the cardiovascular system?

6. What risk factors do you think the average client already knows about?

7. If you suspect your client will only do two things in the area of health promotion for the cardiovascular system, which two things would you recommend first? How would you decide this?

REVIEW QUESTIONS

1. Inspection and palpation for cardiovascular assessment is
   a. an unnecessary concern as it reveals little.
   b. useful in both expected and unexpected findings.

2. Cardiac auscultation areas represent
   a. anatomical location of valves and chambers.
   b. specific locations for best hearing physiological and/or adventitious heart sounds.
   c. an arbitrary designation of pattern for organized auscultation.

3. When taking a routine pulse that seems to be slightly irregular, the nurse should
   a. document findings in the chart as "possibly irregular."
   b. retake the pulse for one full minute.
   c. call the physician.
   d. order a cardiac profile.

4. The term *physiologic splitting* in relation to cardiac auscultation refers to
   a. hearing a slight delay between two simultaneous physiological sounds.
   b. interrupted or split blood flow.
   c. the recommended seesaw pattern of auscultation.

5. A flow murmur occurs with structural defects, high volume (output) demands, or valvular defects.
   a. true
   b. false

Matching:

Cardiac auscultation areas:

6. second left interspace _____
7. second right interspace _____
8. fifth left intercostal space, sternal border _____
9. fifth left intercostal space, midclavicular _____
   a. aortic
   b. pulmonic
   c. tricuspid
   d. mitral

10. Which of the following actions produces the first heart sound S_1?
    a. closing of the mitral and tricuspid valves
    b. closing of the mitral and aortic valves
    c. closing of the aortic and pulmonic valves
    d. closing of the pulmonic and tricuspid valves

11. During auscultation, where is S_2 heard best?
    a. fifth intercostal space at the left sternal border
    b. just under the xiphoid process
    c. at the apex of the heart
    d. left and right second intercostal space

12. Mr. Owen, age 50, came for his yearly health assessment provided by his employer. You are reviewing his heart history. He mentions that he engages in light exercise. At this time you should
    a. record "light exercise."
    b. ask what he means by "light exercise."
    c. record "walks each day."
    d. ask if he makes his own bed each day.

13. Observing the precordium with the client supine *may* allow you to detect clues to heart
    a. heaves or thrusts.
    b. size and symmetry.
    c. conductivity.
    d. consistency.

14. Heart murmurs should be described in relation to loudness, timing, intensity, and radiation. Timing refers to
    a. frequency of occurrence.
    b. occurrence in relation to the cardiac cycle.
    c. time of day the murmur is best heard.
    d. occurrence in relation to physical activity.

15. Bruits are murmurs heard in peripheral vasculature as opposed to the heart itself.
    a. true
    b. false

16. Blood pressure insufficient to maintain adequate perfusion is referred to as
    a. hypotension.
    b. hypertension.
    c. pulsus paradoxus.

17. Which of the following chronic diseases can have serious negative effects on the cardiovascular system? (Circle all that apply.)
    a. cancer
    b. hyperthyroidism
    c. osteoporosis
    d. hypertension
    e. hypotension
    f. Marfan's syndrome
    g. hyperlipidemia

18. Which fetal structures are crucial to the development of the fetus but should resolve shortly after birth?

19. What changes should the examiner expect during cardiac auscultation during inspiration compared to expiration?

20. A client in congestive heart failure will experience several physical assessment changes. List as many factors as you can that are directly identifiable on physical exam.

CASE STUDIES

1. Shondra, a 27-year-old mother, brings Henry, her 2-year-old son, in for his well-child assessment. He is meeting all developmental criteria and taking a good variety of foods. He seems to have little appetite, though he appears interested in his food. Henry is at the 40th percentile for height and weight, though his parents are a bit taller than average height. Henry is friendly and interested in play but is frequently found watching his siblings rather than playing. He often goes off to rest or nap on his own.

   - What family history will be important to know?

   - What birth history is important?

   - What physical assessment factors relative to cardiovascular assessment do you need?

2. Bert Mason, age 73, has come to your primary care clinic complaining of a cough. He gives a good history of a non-productive cough that seems to "come and go." Lately, however, he says it's been pretty persistent. He vowed to be a little more active to see if the cough would clear but has noticed that it grows worse with his increased activity. He also becomes tired more easily. He thinks that his tiredness is related to the fact that he's been awakening two or more times per night to void, and sometimes he feels "almost smothered." Bert's general health history is relatively benign, with only mild COPD as a chronic condition. He takes very little medication, reads a great deal, and plays cards with friends at the senior center. Lately, it almost seems to be too much trouble to get up and go to the activities at the center.

   On general survey, Bert is an erect older male, sallow complected, alert, and focused well on the conversation. You hear what might be an occasional soft wheeze as he leans forward to talk with you.

   - What additional history would you wish? Psychosocial? Past medical? Present problem?

   - What physical assessments would you perform? List all procedures you would accomplish.

CLINICAL ACTIVITIES

In private, assume a comfortable reclining position and assess your heart, its borders, and its characteristic sounds.

- Palpate the PMI (point of maximum impulse), observing for thrills or heaves.
- Auscultate the classic auscultatory areas, first with the diaphragm, then with the bell.
- Note the rhythm, then the sounds themselves.
- Which is loudest in which location?
- Spend time just listening to the heart.
- Notice how its cadence changes as you inspire, then exhale, and then hold your breath.
- Once comfortable with the heart sounds and minor distractions such as hair and fabric against your stethoscope, proceed to assess another person.

Perform a complete cardiac history and physical exam on your lab partner or willing volunteer.

- Use the sample documentation form at the end of the chapter as a guideline.
- Pursue any findings with additional questions or exam procedures.
- Be sure to protect the privacy of your partner or volunteer as you would with a real client. This includes disposing carefully of any written work containing pieces of identifying information.

Sample Documentation Form

Heart and Cardiovascular Assessment

Name: _____ Date: _____

Age: _____ Gender: _____

History

Review of history related to heart and cardiovascular system:

_____

YES/NO   If YES, provide details:

_____

General

☐	☐	Smoking	_____
☐	☐	Fatigue	_____
☐	☐	Overweight/obesity	_____
☐	☐	Level of stress	_____
☐	☐	Exercise	_____
☐	☐	Alcohol consumption	_____
☐	☐	Diet	_____
☐	☐	Diabetes mellitus	_____

Cardiovascular

☐	☐	Cardiac disease history	_____
☐	☐	Chest pain or tightness	_____
☐	☐	Irregular heartbeat	_____
☐	☐	Unexplained dizziness	_____
☐	☐	Blood pressure problems	_____
☐	☐	Shortness of breath	_____
☐	☐	Orthopnea	_____
☐	☐	Cough	_____
☐	☐	Edema or cold hands or feet	_____
☐	☐	Color changes/hands	_____
☐	☐	Color changes/lower legs or feet	_____
☐	☐	Swelling/ankles or legs	_____
☐	☐	Nocturia	_____

Focused symptom analysis of current problem:

Reason for visit: _____

_____

Character: _____

Onset: _____

Duration: _____

Location: _____

Severity: _____

Associated problems: _____

Efforts to treat: _____

Current medications (note, hormones):

_____

Social history (fitness/exercise, stress reduction, nutrition):

_____

_____

_____

Sleep/rest patterns: _____

_____

Family history of problems relating to the heart or cardiovascular system (especially cardiac arrest), or diabetes mellitus:

_____

_____

_____

Physical Assessment
Height and weight:

Height in inches: _____ Weight in pounds: _____ BMI: _____

		TIME OF ASSESSMENT			
Hour		a.m. p.m.	a.m. p.m.	a.m. p.m.	a.m. p.m.
Pulse	R = Radial A = Apical Rhythm				
Right	BP Systolic Diastolic				
Left	BP Systolic Diastolic				

Cardiovascular System:
Inspection and Palpation

General characteristics (skin color, temperature and tone, cyanosis, nail clubbing or spooning, venous stasis): _____

_____

Anterior chest (color, symmetry, contour, scars, venous pattern, apical impulse, pulsations/thrills/heaves): _____

_____

Carotid and jugular vessels (pulsations, distention): _____

Abdominal vessels (aorta, iliac, renal pulsations): _____

Peripheral circulation (arms, legs, hands, and feet for temperature, color and pulses, ulcers and skin condition): _____

_____

Auscultation (with diaphragm and bell):

All cardiac locations (rate, rhythm, S_1, S_2, note any extra sounds, splits, murmurs):

Aortic: _____

Pulmonic: _____

Tricuspid: _____

Mitral: _____

Auscultate arteries for bruits.

Carotid: _____

Abdominal aorta: _____

Iliac arteries: _____

Renal arteries: _____

Analysis:

_____

_____

_____

_____

Nursing diagnoses: _____

_____

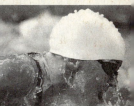

OVERVIEW

The heart and peripheral vasculature are extensions of each other. Any separation is simply a convenient organizational way to consider a complex system. That which affects one will directly affect the other. Consequently, most historical questions for the heart will provide useful information for both ends of the system. An additional cluster of questions and the extended physical exams, then, bestow deeper knowledge of the health and functioning of the complete system.

ASSIGNMENT

CD-ROM content: Chapter 18, especially animations
Companion website: www.prenhall.com/damico, Chapter 18

VOCABULARY EXERCISE

After completing the reading assignment, you should be able to define the **key terms** listed below. Refer back to the page number from the main text for help.

Allen's test, 486
Arterial aneurysm, 502
Arterial insufficiency, 502
Arteries, 477
Bruit, 489
Capillaries, 478
Clubbing, 489
Edema, 489
Epitrochlear node, 479
Homans' sign, 495

Lymph, 478
Lymph nodes, 478
Lymphatic vessels, 478
Manual compression test, 486
Peripheral vascular system, 477
Pulse, 477
Raynaud's disease, 504
Varicosities, 493
Veins, 478
Venous insufficiency, 483

ANATOMY EXERCISES

1. Label all lines on main arteries.

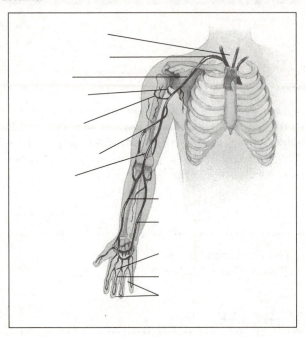

Figure 18–1

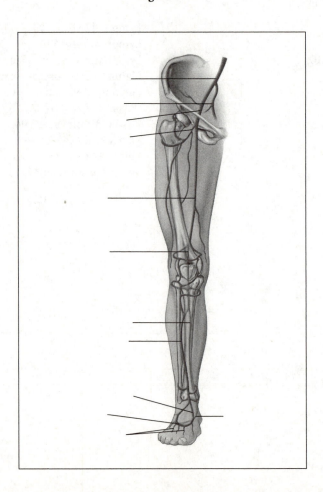

Figure 18–2

2. On both figures, locate and label points that you would use for assessment of pulses.

3. On Figure 18–1 indicate likely places you might use to administer IV therapy.

4. Label lines indicating main lymph nodes and channels.

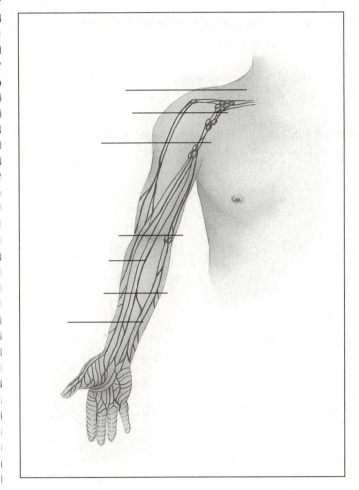

Figure 18–3

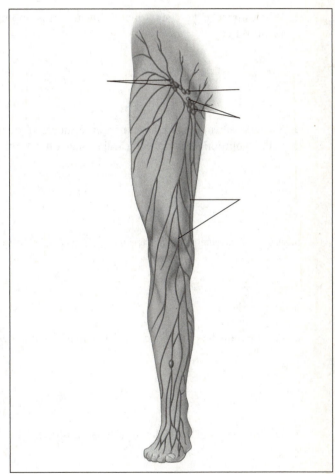

Figure 18–4

5. Why is it important to be able to locate lymph nodes? What client problems might make it important for you to assess and then document these nodes?

STUDY FOCUS

1. List three chronic conditions that are of great risk to the peripheral cardiovascular system.

2. After reading your chapter information, what can you identify as the most damaging behaviors in relation to cardiovascular health?

3. When measuring a client's blood pressure, it is important to document the client's position during measurement. Why?

4. Skin assessment is a significant part of cardiovascular assessment. What negative skin findings might be associated with compromised peripheral cardiovascular function?

5. Is edema associated with arterial or venous compromise?

6. What parameters should be measured, then documented, when assessing a pulse?

7. List the signs and symptoms of arterial insufficiency.

REVIEW QUESTIONS

1. The difference in rate, if any, between apical and peripheral pulse is referred to as
   a. pulse pressure.
   b. pulse deficit.
   c. insignificant if less than 15 beats per minute.
   d. venous insufficiency.

2. The auscultatory method of assessing blood pressure *always* involves
   a. intermittent obliteration of an artery.
   b. the brachial artery.
   c. use of a stethoscope.
   d. listening for at least three changes in the sound of the pulse.

3. In blood pressure assessment, a too large/wide cuff will yield falsely _____ readings.
   a. high
   b. low

4. Palpating the artery during cuff inflation for obliteration of pulse prior to blood pressure measurement will
   a. elevate the systolic measurement.
   b. yield a palpated systolic measurement.
   c. elevate the diastolic measurement.
   d. invalidate the second reading due to arterial compression.

5. Bruits are murmurs heard in peripheral vasculature as opposed to the heart itself.
   a. true
   b. false

6. Peripheral pulses, when compared to the apical pulse, should be identical in all of the following except
   a. rate.
   b. rhythm.
   c. amplitude.
   d. all should be equal.

7. To rate the amplitude (or quality) of a pulse as a 2/4 is to indicate the pulse is
   a. half of the expected amplitude.
   b. in a range of 2 to 4.
   c. 2 on a scale of 0 to 4.
   d. none of the above.

8. Blood pressure insufficient to maintain adequate perfusion is referred to as
   a. hypotension.
   b. hypertension.
   c. pulsus paradoxus.

9. Peripheral circulatory insufficiency resulting in the following symptoms: pain on use (exercise), ulcers on tips of extremities, pallor, cyanosis, and pain unrelieved by elevation of the extremity, is
   a. arterial.
   b. venous.

10. Range of normal blood pressure is 10 mm Hg higher when using the aneroid rather than the mercury manometer.
    a. true
    b. false

11. A difference of more than 10 mm Hg in blood pressure between the right and left arm is
    a. indicative of a possible circulatory obstruction.
    b. unremarkable.

c. called a negative Allen test.
d. related to position.

12. Assessment of the carotid arteries should include
    a. simultaneous palpation of the right and left artery.
    b. auscultation for bruit.
    c. measurement of distention of vessels above the clavicle.
    d. assessment of overlying skin.

13. Examination of the fingers and their nails yields information relative to (circle all that apply)
    a. respiratory status.
    b. cardiovascular status.
    c. renal compromise.
    d. nutritional health.

14. The epitrochlear node is located _____.

15. Skin color in the pretibial area is affected by poor _____.

16. A positive Homans' sign could be indicative of a deep vein thrombosis. It could also indicate _____ or _____.

17. Findings of poor color, thickened toenails, and altered sensation in the toes would require careful assessment of which pulses?

18. Sensory loss in fingers and/or toes is associated with (circle all that apply)
    a. poor arterial circulation.
    b. peripheral neuropathy.
    c. pulsus paradoxus.
    d. venous insufficiency.
    e. Raynaud's disease.

19. Difference in amplitude between right and left pulses indicates _____.

20. Signs and symptoms of deep vein thrombosis include _____, _____, _____, and _____.

21. Edema may be
    a. local.
    b. regional.
    c. generalized.
    d. all of the above.

CASE STUDY

1. Allen, age 62, has been making an effort to be a bit more active. He has been trying to increase his walking on a daily basis and has been keeping a diary about the actual distance. Reviewing his diary, he finds that he is losing ground rather than increasing his distance. He is walking until his legs begin to ache and then reluctantly turning back to rest. He finds he is somewhat breathless as well.

   - What specifics about his reason for seeking healthcare do you need to know?

   - What are his two main symptoms?

   - What might you find on skin assessment of Allen's lower extremities?

   - What physical assessment findings would cause you to recommend that Allen not continue to push for an increase in walking distance at this time?

   - What special tests could you perform to assess Allen's circulation?

   - What nursing diagnoses might apply at this time to Allen?

CLINICAL ACTIVITIES

Perform a complete peripheral vascular history and physical exam on your lab partner or willing volunteer.

- Use the sample documentation form at the end of the chapter as guideline.
- Pursue any findings with additional questions or exam procedures.

▶ Be sure to protect the privacy of your partner or volunteer as you would with a real client. This includes disposing carefully of any written work containing pieces of identifying information. In assessing circulation there is always the possibility of lesions or ulcers on extremities. If such lesions are observed, be sure to implement Standard Precautions for any drainage.

Sample Documentation Form

Peripheral Vascular

Name: _____ Date: _____

Age: _____ Gender: _____

Review of history related to the current visit:

Focused symptom analysis of current problem:

    Reason for visit: _____

    _____

    Character: _____

    Onset: _____

    Duration: _____

    Location: _____

    Severity: _____

    Associated problems: _____

    Efforts to treat: _____

History

Review of history related to the peripheral vascular system:

YES/NO   *If YES, provide details:*

☐ ☐   Pain or cold in hands or feet   _____

☐ ☐   Color changes in hands   _____

☐ ☐   Pain or color changes in lower legs or feet _____

☐ ☐   Swelling in ankles or legs   _____

☐ ☐   Ulcers on ankles   _____

☐ ☐   Cardiac disease   _____

☐ ☐   Diabetes   _____

☐ ☐   Circulatory problems   _____

☐ ☐   Blood pressure problems   _____

Current medications: _____

_____

Family history (blood pressure, circulatory problems, or diabetes mellitus): _____

_____

_____

Physical Assessment

Peripheral Perfusion: Upper Extremities

Inspection/Palpation

General appearance (skin color, texture, moisture; temperature; hair distribution, intactness; limb symmetry; edema; lesions): _____

_____

_____

Capillary refill (less than 2 seconds): _____

Lymph nodes (upper body): _____

Fingernail base angle (presence of clubbing or spooning): _____

Venous obstruction or insufficiency (erythema and/or cyanosis, thickening, temperature, skin lesions, or shiny skin): _____

Varicose veins: _____

Edema (present or absent—if present, describe severity by degree): _____

1+	mild pitting, slight indentation, no perceptible swelling	3+	deep pitting, indentation remains for a short time, looks swollen
2+	moderate pitting, indentation, subsides rapidly	4+	very deep pitting, indentation lasts for a long time, limb appears swollen

Peripheral Perfusion: Lower Extremities

General appearance (skin color, texture, moisture; temperature; skin intactness; limb symmetry; edema): _____

Toenails: _____

Capillary refill (less than 2 seconds): _____

Lymph nodes (lower body): _____

Venous obstruction or insufficiency (erythema and/or cyanosis, thickening, temperature, skin lesions, or shiny skin): _____

Varicose veins: _____

Edema (present or absent—if present, describe severity by degree): _____

1+	mild pitting, slight indentation, no perceptible swelling	3+	deep pitting, indentation remains for a short time, looks swollen
2+	moderate pitting, indentation, subsides rapidly	4+	very deep pitting, indentation lasts for a long time, limb appears swollen

Blood Pressures

		TIME OF ASSESSMENT			
Hour		a.m. p.m.	a.m. p.m.	a.m. p.m.	a.m. p.m.
	Right				
Blood Pressure	Systolic / Diastolic				
	Left				
Blood Pressure	Systolic / Diastolic				

Pulses

		Pulse Rate/minute	Pulse Rhythm	Pulse Amplitude Absent (0) Thready/weak (1+) Normal (2+) Increased (3+) Bounding (4+)
Carotid	Right			
	Left			
Brachial	Right			
	Left			
Radial	Right			
	Left			
Femoral	Right			
	Left			
Popliteal	Right			
	Left			
Dorsalis pedis	Right			
	Left			
Posterior tibial	Right			
	Left			

Note if Doppler is needed to identify pulse: _____

Additional Tests:

Allen test (color return): _____

Manual compression test: _____

Homans' sign: _____

Analysis:

_____

_____

_____

Nursing diagnoses: _____

_____

19 Abdomen

OVERVIEW

The abdomen seems quite unremarkable at casual inspection. The professional nurse knows, however, that it contains organs of such importance that life is not possible should any one of them fail. This most significant array of physiology demands a meticulous and complex history and a physical assessment that includes all vital organs. Relevant history includes not only past medical and present functioning, but also diet and many lifestyle behaviors such as substance abuse and communicable disease exposure. Assessment techniques vary here too, with auscultation following inspection so that the bowel is assessed before it is stimulated by percussion or palpation. In the female of childbearing years, it is most important to assess the possibility of pregnancy before any assessment or treatment takes place.

ASSIGNMENT

CD-ROM content: Chapter 19, especially clinical spotlight videos
Companion website: www.prenhall.com/damico, Chapter 19

VOCABULARY EXERCISE

After completing the reading assignment, you should be able to define the **key terms** listed below. Refer back to the page number from the main text for help.

Abdomen, 511
Accessory digestive organs, 513
Alimentary canal, 511
Anorexia nervosa, 548
Ascites, 541
Blumberg's sign, 540
Bruit, 532
Dysphagia, 548
Esophagitis, 549
Friction rub, 532

Hernia, 546
Malnutrition, 548
Mapping, 515
Obesity, 548
Overweight, 548
Peritoneum, 513
Peritonitis, 549
Referred pain, 544
Striae, 531

ANATOMY EXERCISES

1. Using the lines provided label the various structures of the abdomen.

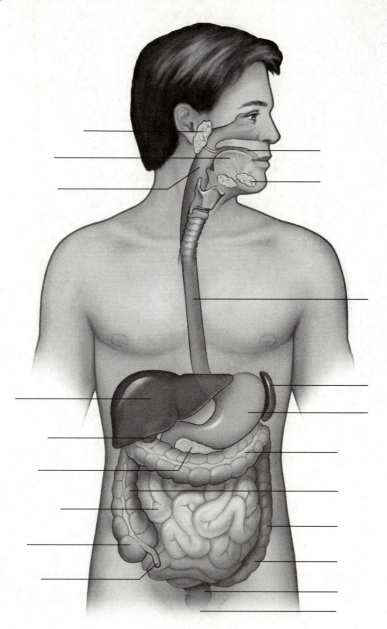

Figure 19–1

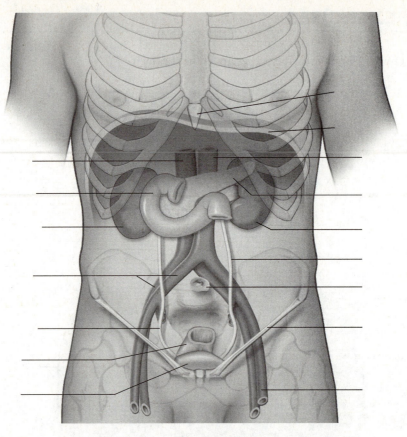

Figure 19–2

2. Identify the organs of the abdomen that have bony protection. Identify the major vessels in the abdomen that do not have bony protection.

3. Label all anatomical structures.

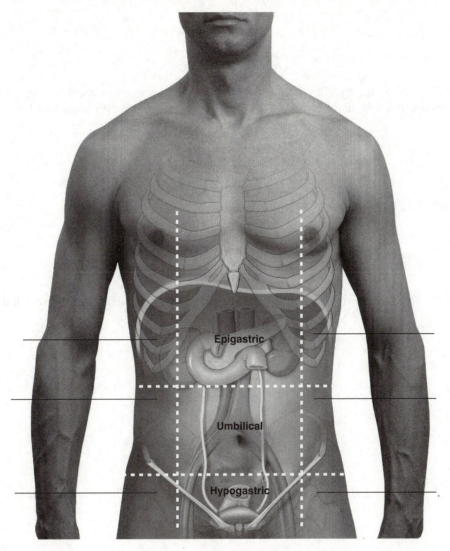

Epigastric

Umbilical

Hypogastric

Figure 19–3

4. This map of the abdomen is very useful for documenting your findings, or client indications of the location of pain. Label organs in each of the regions indicated.

STUDY FOCUS

1. What are the two extremes of malnutrition? Is one any more dangerous than the other?

2. What general advice can the nurse give a client who is complaining of constipation? In exploring the symptom history of constipation, what is one complaint that may be indicative of a more serious problem?

3. List three causes of protuberant abdomen.

4. What are high-risk behaviors for liver health? What are some adventitious signs in assessment of the liver?

5. What are the physical assessment signs of peritoneal irritation?

6. Pain in the left shoulder could be associated with what abdominal organ? This pain would be called _____ pain.

7. Hernia is the protrusion of the contents of one body cavity into another, or to the exterior. What parts of the abdomen could give rise to hernia?

REVIEW QUESTIONS

1. Prior to abdominal exam, the examiner should
   a. ascertain the client's HIV status.
   b. have the client empty his or her bladder.
   c. double glove.
   d. completely disrobe the client.

2. When examining a client with tense abdominal musculature, a helpful technique is to have the client
   a. hold his or her breath.
   b. sit upright.
   c. flex his or her knees.
   d. raise his or her head off the pillow.

3. Your client is diagnosed with duodenal ulcer and is complaining of thoracic back pain. A likely explanation is that the client is experiencing
   a. referred pain.
   b. rebound tenderness.
   c. Cullen's sign.
   d. striae.

4. After thorough inspection of the abdomen, the next assessment step is to
   a. percuss.
   b. palpate.
   c. auscultate.
   d. perform a rectal exam.

5. To establish absence of bowel sounds, one must listen continuously for
   a. 30 seconds.
   b. 1 minute.
   c. 3 minutes.
   d. 5 minutes.

True or False: These factors would put a client at *specific* risk for abdominal pathology. Answer true or false by using the letter a for true and the letter b for false.

6. more than moderate alcohol intake _____

7. cocaine abuse _____

8. a highly spicy diet _____

9. smoking _____

10. IV drug abuse _____

11. sustained travel to third world countries _____

12. Assessment of the abdomen evaluates in part _____ status. (Circle all that apply.)
    a. cardiovascular
    b. bowel
    c. skin
    d. neurologic
    e. renal

13. Indirect abdominal percussion should allow identification of
    a. liver, spleen, and stomach.
    b. liver, gallbladder, and uterus.
    c. spleen, stomach, and rectum.
    d. uterus, kidneys, and liver.

14. Percussion in the right midclavicular line, below the level of the umbilicus and continuing upward, is a correct technique for locating the
    a. lower liver border.
    b. upper right kidney border.

   c. medial border of the spleen.
   d. descending aorta.

15. Pain is a clear indication of abdominal pathology.
    a. true
    b. false

16. Dysphasia is another name for heartburn.
    a. true
    b. false

17. Mild to moderate visible peristalsis and abdominal pulsation can be expected findings in a very thin client.
    a. true
    b. false

18. Costovertebral angle tenderness can be a sign of a problem with the
    a. colon.
    b. gallbladder.
    c. kidney(s).
    d. liver.

19. Before beginning assessment of the abdomen on a female, it is most important to
    a. ensure privacy.
    b. determine possibility of pregnancy.
    c. ask about sexually transmitted disease.
    d. discover if she is ticklish.

20. Dullness to percussion would occur over
    a. solid tumor.
    b. empty bladder.
    c. gaseous distention.
    d. pelvic bones.

21. A client complaining of constipation should be
    a. counseled about diet and exercise.
    b. advised to increase fluid intake.
    c. questioned about his or her definition of constipation.
    d. examined for hemorrhoids.

22. Ascites is an adventitious collection of fluid in the abdomen discernible on percussion.
    a. true
    b. false

23. A urine-filled bladder is _____ to percussion, while an empty bladder is _____.
    a. dull, unavailable to percussion
    b. resonant, flat
    c. tympanic, dull

24. Adventitious findings related to the spleen include
   a. spleen is dull to percussion.
   b. visible peristalsis.
   c. splenic descent is less than 4 cm.
   d. spleen is palpable below T_{10} in the mid-axillary line.

25. During abdominal palpation, the examiner becomes aware of a bulging in the mid left upper quadrant. Likely this is
   a. umbilical hernia.
   b. abdominal aorta.
   c. inguinal hernia.
   d. ascites.

CASE STUDIES

1. Hank, a 21-year-old college student, presents at the emergency room complaining of copious vomiting of approximately 2 days duration. He admits to considerable alcohol intake at a "nice oyster bar" to celebrate his 21st birthday. He says the vomiting is subsiding somewhat but now he feels sick all over, achy, and feverish. He says he's never had a hangover like this before.

- What immediate assessment do you want to do?

- Outline a symptom history for the vomiting.

- Regardless of final diagnosis, what dangers are there for Hank if the vomiting continues?

- What general physical assessment is in order?

- What abdominal findings are possible given his symptoms?

- What personal social history is essential?

- Which nursing diagnoses are appropriate to Hank at this time?

2. Martha is a 42-year-old female who presents complaining of lack of appetite, difficulty swallowing, and an irritating cough. She denies recent upper respiratory infection or flu symptoms. She states that sometimes she awakens shortly after falling asleep at night with a feeling of indigestion, even though she has eaten lightly. She denies history of gastrointestinal pathology, surgery, or exposure to anyone actively ill.

- What immediate physical assessment do you want to do?

- Outline a symptom history for the cough, lack of appetite, and the dysphagia.

- What specific medical history would you wish?

- What personal social history would you wish?

- What specific signs would you look for on physical assessment?

- What nursing diagnosis might apply to Martha?

CLINICAL ACTIVITIES

Field Trip

Take a field trip to your neighborhood pharmacy and visit the selection of medications related to the gastrointestinal system.

- Read labels on laxatives, antidiarrheals, antiemetics, antacids, proton pump inhibitors, appetite suppressants, and so on.
- Be aware of what clients may be using to self-medicate before they seek professional care.

Abdominal Exam

With your nursing lab partner or willing volunteer, take a thorough history of the abdominal organs and the lifestyle behaviors affecting them.

- Let the history direct any special attention needed to specific areas.

- Have your client empty his or her bladder.
- Be sure to provide privacy for your client and to have gloves handy for your use should there be any possibility of exposure to body fluids.
- For the ticklish client, be sure to warm your hands and try to maintain some physical contact consistently, rather than touching intermittently. Use the sample documentation form at the end of this chapter as a guideline.

In a true clinical setting,

- Have specimen collection apparatus available before beginning the exam.
- Be sure to protect yourself and all clinical surfaces from exposure to body fluids by implementing Standard Precautions. Review these in Appendices B and C in your text.

Sample Documentation Form

Abdomen and Gastrointestinal Assessment

Name: _____ Date: _____

Age: _____ Gender: _____

_____

Focused symptom analysis of current problem:

Reason for visit: _____

_____

Character: _____

Onset: _____

Duration: _____

Location: _____

Severity: _____

Associated problems: _____

Efforts to treat: _____

Current medications: _____

_____

History

For female clients, last menstrual period: _____

Review of history related to abdomen and gastrointestinal system:

_____

YES/NO   If YES, provide details:

_____

Dietary

☐ ☐   Recent weight change   _____

☐ ☐   Concerned about weight   _____

☐ ☐   Appetite change   _____

☐ ☐   Food allergies or intolerances _____

☐ ☐   On special diet at present   _____

☐ ☐   Use of food supplements   _____

☐ ☐   Use of weight-controlling drugs _____

☐ ☐   Eating disorders   _____

Dietary recall, if not previously done (see Chapter 9):

Gastrointestinal System

☐ ☐   Gastrointestinal, hepatic,
        gallbladder, pancreatic disease _____

☐ ☐   Abdominal surgeries   _____

☐ ☐   Diabetes   _____

☐ ☐   Difficulty swallowing   _____

☐ ☐   Change in bowel habits   _____

☐ ☐   Indigestion   _____

☐ ☐   Burping/increased gas   _____

☐	☐	Heartburn or gastric reflux
☐	☐	Abdominal pain
☐	☐	Nausea, vomiting, diarrhea
☐	☐	Flatulence or increased gas
☐	☐	Substance abuse (alcohol, other drugs)

Stools

☐	☐	Difficulty with bowel movements
☐	☐	Diarrhea/constipation
☐	☐	Consistency of stools
☐	☐	Fecal incontinence
☐	☐	Stool characteristics
☐	☐	Frequency of bowel movements
☐	☐	Color of stools

Liver

☐	☐	Jaundice
☐	☐	Diarrhea
☐	☐	Color of urine
☐	☐	Immunizations
☐	☐	Substance abuse

Family history of problems related to the gastrointestinal system, diabetes: _____
_____

Physical Assessment

Height and Weight

Height in inches: _____   Weight in pounds: _____   BMI: _____

Abdomen:

Inspection

General characteristics (color, symmetry, contour, scars, venous pattern, pulsations, peristalsis, umbilicus, hernia; identify any enteral tubes):

_____
_____
_____

Auscultation

General characteristics (four quadrant characteristics of bowel sounds—presence, characteristics, frequency): _____

_____
_____

Abdominal vascular system for bruits (aorta, iliac, renal arteries):_____

_____

Percussion

General characteristics (four quadrant characteristics of abdominal tones over small and large intestine, liver, and gastric bubble): _____

_____

_____

Liver (location, liver span, and borders): _____

_____

Spleen (location, spleen location, span, and borders): _____

_____

Palpation

General characteristics (four quadrant characteristics of abdomen using light and deep palpation. Note muscle tone, tenderness, pain, discomfort, lumps and/or masses, inguinal lymph nodes, femoral pulses): _____

_____

_____

Liver (location, liver span, and borders): _____

Spleen (location, spleen location, span, and borders): _____

_____

Special Evaluation Procedures

Rebound tenderness (pain reported following rapid removal of hand from position of deep palpation): _____

_____

Psoas sign (hip flexion from supine position causes pain): _____

_____

Murphy's sign (palpate liver; if gallbladder descends to meet examiner's fingers, the client has abrupt disruption of inspiration): _____

Special Findings

Ascites: _____

Enteral tubes (location, condition): _____

Analysis:

_____

_____

_____

Nursing diagnoses: _____

_____

Urinary System 20

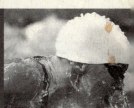

OVERVIEW

The urinary system is renowned as a waste disposal system, but it plays a great role in conservation as well. A healthy system conserves fluid, electrolytes, proteins, and blood cells. The system especially reflects functioning in the cardiovascular, reproductive, and endocrine systems.

Clients can usually give a very objective history of urinary habits and occurrences. Reports about urgency, bed-wetting, incontinence, backaches, and painful urination give significant information about the urinary system and other interdependent systems. Examination of the system reveals local integrity and response to the functioning of other systems.

ASSIGNMENT

CD-ROM content: Chapter 20, especially clinical spotlight videos
Companion website: www.prenhall.com/damico, Chapter 20

VOCABULARY EXERCISE

After completing the reading assignment, you should be able to define the **key terms** listed below. Refer back to the page number from the main text for help.

Calculi, 560
Cortex, 555
Costovertebral angle, 557
Dysreflexia, 577
Enuresis, 566
Glomeruli, 555
Hematuria, 572
Incontinence, 577

Kidneys, 555
Medulla, 555
Nocturia, 560
Oliguria, 572
Ureters, 557
Urethra, 557
Urinary retention, 577

ANATOMY EXERCISES

1. Label all anatomical structures.

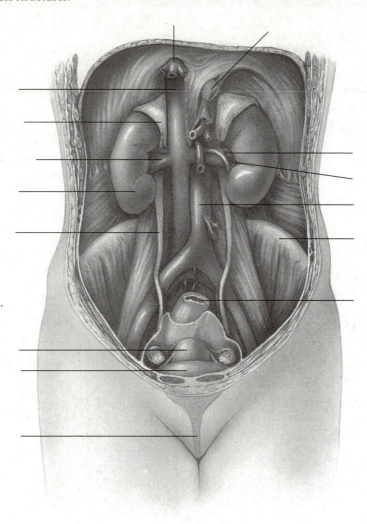

Figure 20–1

2. Note the major blood vessels in close proximity to the kidneys (Figure 20–1). Note also the long slender ureters that travel to the bladder. How difficult would it be to block a ureter?

3. Label all anatomical structures.

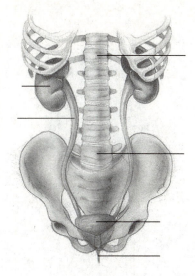

Figure 20–2

4. Looking at Figure 20–2, where do you see opportunities for obstruction in the urinary tract?

5. Label all structures of the kidney.

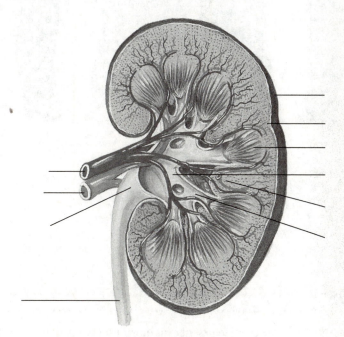

Figure 20–3

6. Label kidneys and CVA.

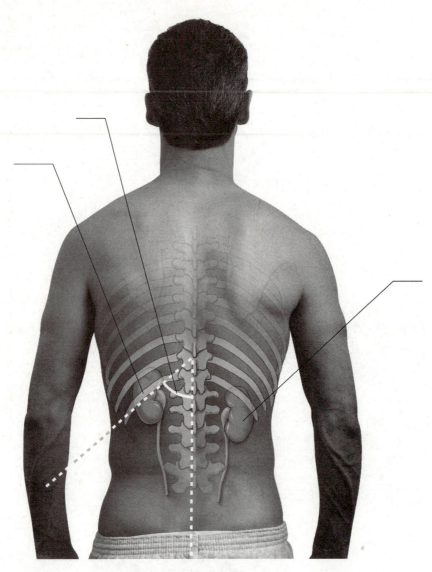

Figure 20–4

STUDY FOCUS

1. In taking a history, the nurse asks the client to describe his or her usual urinary habits. Is there a standard to which the client's pattern can be compared? What are the physiological factors that affect the frequency and amount of voiding? Is there a minimum of urinary output per day?

2. Control of voiding is developmentally dependent. At what age is it reasonable to expect voluntary urinary control?

3. Diabetes and hypertension are severe threats to the urinary system. What is the specific mechanism by which diabetes and hypertension affect the urinary system?

4. What urinary symptoms would indicate a possible cardiovascular malfunction?

5. List specific health protection measures that can be taken to avoid risk to the urinary system.

6. Fist or blunt percussion to the kidney is an accepted technique of assessment. What response to this technique would indicate possible pathology of the kidney? Explain why this response occurs in the state of infection or inflammation.

7. On general survey, what assessment factors might the nurse see in a client with chronic kidney disease?

REVIEW QUESTIONS

1. A urine-filled bladder is _____ to percussion, while an empty bladder is _____.
   a. dull, unavailable to percussion
   b. resonant, flat
   c. tympanic, dull

2. Urinary frequency may indicate (circle all that apply)
   a. overdistention of the bladder.
   b. acute kidney failure.
   c. incomplete emptying of the bladder.
   d. fluid retention.

3. The usual amount of urine voided in a typical voiding five to six times per day for an adult under routine intake patterns is
   a. 100 to 400 ml.
   b. 500 ml.
   c. 60 ml per hour.

4. Nocturia may result from
   a. normal aging patterns.
   b. congestive heart failure.
   c. lack of bladder control.
   d. depression.
   e. a and b.

5. Risks to the urinary tract from diabetes include (circle all that apply)
   a. glycosuria.
   b. bacterial infection.
   c. yeast infection.
   d. proteinuria.
   e. renal calculi.

6. Risks to the urinary tract from hypertension include (circle all that apply)
   a. glycosuria.
   b. bacterial infection.
   c. yeast infection.
   d. proteinuria.
   e. renal calculi.

7. List at least four common complaints from a client with a urinary tract infection.

8. List at least four common physical assessment findings in a client with a urinary infection.

9. In the male client, difficulty initiating or maintaining a urine stream may be related to (circle all that apply)
   a. urinary tract infection.
   b. kidney infection.
   c. prostate enlargement.
   d. prostate infection or inflammation.
   e. glycosuria.

10. The relationship of low-set ears and possible kidney problems is one of
    a. history of infection.
    b. fetal development.
    c. irrationality.
    d. a recognized syndrome.

11. A common but expected change in urinary pattern for the pregnant female is increased.
    a. amounts of voided urine.
    b. specific gravity of urine.
    c. frequency of urination.
    d. itching and possible burning on voiding.

12. On abdominal inspection, it may be possible to identify the full urinary bladder in a client who is 5′5″ tall and weighs 110 lbs.
    a. true
    b. false

Matching: Match the conditions listed after question 16 with the appropriate description.

13. _____ small to no urine output

14. _____ excessive voiding at night

15. _____ increased frequency of voiding

16. _____ visible blood in urine
    a. polyuria
    b. oliguria
    c. hematuria
    d. nocturia

17. Fluid retention is an expected sign with
    a. bladder infection.
    b. kidney failure.
    c. diabetes.
    d. urinary tract infection.

CASE STUDIES

Olivia is a nurse for the residents of a long-term care facility. Incontinence is a common but serious problem for residents. It can increase the discomfort of clients with limited mobility, increase the risk of infection, and decrease the quality of life. Chapter 20 lists five types of incontinence. Following are four clients and a brief description of their situations. Indicate which of the five types of incontinence each might be found to have. Then indicate what nursing actions might be helpful for each.

1. Mrs. Sabido is 84 years old and somewhat confused. She is easily cued by objects, such as her walker, her clothing, and so on. She is not able to plan nor can she remember things for more than a few seconds. She often has accidents while walking in the halls.

   Likely type of incontinence:

   Nursing intervention related to incontinence:

How would this be expressed as a nursing diagnosis?

2. Harry is a 34-year-old quadriplegic who has been in care for several years. He is alert but not involved in any activities. He sometimes uses an indwelling catheter but often simply stays in his room, and a caregiver changes his clothing if he becomes wet.

   Likely type of incontinence:

   Nursing intervention related to incontinence:

   Applicable nursing diagnosis:

3. Angel Garner is an 84-year-old resident who is very social. She especially loves to sing and happily joins any group activity that involves singing. Often, during a stirring performance, she finds herself wet. For this reason she is considering dropping out of choir.

   Likely type of incontinence:

   Nursing intervention related to incontinence:

   Applicable nursing diagnosis:

4. Miss Viola, 86 years of age, is very fragile, but most of the day she can keep up with her voiding needs. She is very social and looks forward to meals as an opportunity to visit. She eats very little but will often sit and drink tea and visit for as long as she can capture a companion. Many times, she becomes tearful in the dining room because she has had an accident or is fearful that she will do so.

Likely type of incontinence:

Nursing intervention related to incontinence:

Nursing diagnosis:

CLINICAL ACTIVITIES

Perform a complete urinary history and physical assessment on your lab partner or willing volunteer. Use the sample documentation form at the end of this chapter as a guideline. Pursue any findings with additional questions or assessment procedures. Be sure to protect the privacy of your partner or volunteer as you would with a real client. This includes deleting of any written work containing pieces of identifying information.

In a clinical experience, read your client's chart and look for a urinalysis report. If there are any abnormal findings, look for observable symptoms that may be associated with these findings.

Sample Documentation Form

Urinary System

Name: _____   Date: _____

Age: _____   Gender: _____

Review of history related to urinary system:

_____

YES/NO   If YES, provide details:
_____

☐ ☐   Kidney disease   _____

☐ ☐   Bladder infection   _____

☐ ☐   Cancer history   _____

☐ ☐   Change urinary patterns   _____

☐ ☐   Congenital urinary problems   _____

☐ ☐   Bladder control   _____

☐ ☐   Problems with urine stream   _____

☐ ☐   Urinary frequency   _____

☐ ☐   Infection   _____

☐ ☐   Sexually transmitted disease
        (STD) history   _____

☐ ☐   Prostate problems   _____

☐ ☐   Edema   _____

☐ ☐   Diabetes   _____

Females, last menstrual period: _____

Problem Statement

Focused symptom analysis of current problem:

Reason for visit: _____

_____

Character: _____

Onset: _____

Duration: _____

Location: _____

Severity: _____

Associated problems: _____

Efforts to treat: _____

Physical Assessment

Inspection

Skin (color, odor): _____

Urinary meatus (location, inflammation, discharge): _____

Abdomen (symmetry, contour, scars, enteral tubes, lesions, suprapubic distention): _____

_____

Auscultation

Renal arteries (for bruits): _____

Palpation

Costovertebral angle (symmetry, tenderness): _____

Kidney palpation (abdominal/flank palpation to identify size and placement, right and left):

_____

Urinary bladder palpation (size, symmetry, tenderness): _____

Percussion

Costovertebral angles (first percussion for tenderness): _____

_____

Abdomen (indirect percussion of the bladder): _____

Analysis: _____

_____

_____

Nursing diagnosis: _____

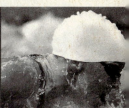

OVERVIEW

Most of us think of reproductive activities as production of offspring and sexual pleasure, and certainly this is true. But reproductive functioning is equally critical to reproducing life-sustaining processes, such as tissue maintenance, absorption of critical elements, and generation and maintenance of sexual characteristics. Hormones associated with reproductive functions are responsible for many additional aspects of life. Problems in this system evidence themselves in biological, psychosocial, and psychological aspects of living. Consequently, the history the nurse takes and the physical assessment that is performed are of equal and immense importance. An additional consideration is that there may be some reluctance on the part of a client to discuss aspects of the reproductive system. By taking care to establish a rapport and to initiate discussion in a comfortable and accepting manner, the nurse can elicit a more comprehensive and directive history than might have been otherwise possible.

ASSIGNMENT

CD-ROM content: Chapter 21, especially clinical spotlight video
Companion website: www.prenhall.com/damico, Chapter 21

VOCABULARY EXERCISE

After completing the reading assignment, you should be able to define the **key terms** listed below. Refer back to the page number from the main text for help.

Anus, 586
Bulbourethral glands, 586
Cremasteric reflex, 604
Epididymis, 585
Epididymitis, 595
Epispadias, 586
Hypospadias, 586
Inguinal hernia, 586
Orchitis, 602
Penis, 586
Perineum, 586
Peyronie's disease, 592

Phimosis, 586
Prostate gland, 586
Scrotum, 583
Seminal vesicles, 585
Smegma, 600
Spermatic cord, 585
Spermatocele, 602
Testes, 584
Urethra, 585
Urethral stricture, 601
Varicocele, 604

ANATOMY EXERCISES

1. Label all anatomical structures.

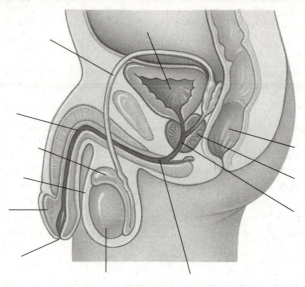

Figure 21–1

Note the relationship of the prostate to the rectum. Remember that you will evaluate the posterior aspect of the prostate through the anterior rectal wall on digital exam.

2. Label all anatomical structures.

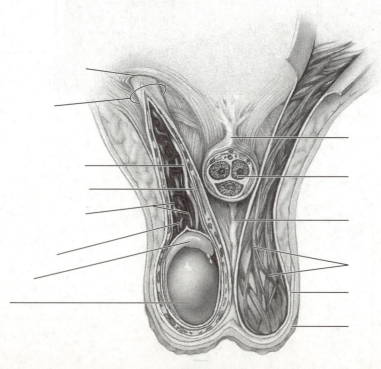

Figure 21–2

3. Note the vertical alignment of the reproductive apparatus. Visualize your soft tissue assessment from the testes up to the inguinal ring. Do you think the epididymis could be easily mistaken for an abnormal growth on the testes if one lacked the anatomical knowledge?

4. Label all anatomical structures.

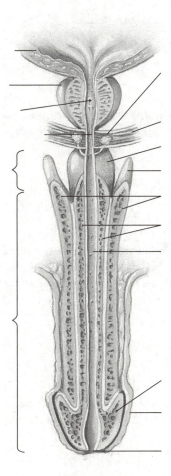

Figure 21–3

5. As you identify structures, think about the process of catheterization. Which structures would be contacted during a catheterization? Which structures if swollen or inflamed might impede the procedure?

STUDY FOCUS

1. Cultural and developmental influences can significantly affect the conducting of a history of the reproductive system. Name two cultural and two developmental factors that might compromise the taking of a reproductive history. (See Chapters 3 and 4 in addition to Chapter 21 in your text for additional ideas.)

2. Two types of male reproductive cancers are more common among Caucasians than among other races. They are _____ and _____.

3. The original rationale for male circumcision was to improve hygiene and subsequently reduce infection and cancer. What is the current information on this rationale? What is the current rate of male circumcision in the United States?

4. During a focused interview for male reproductive history, the nurse will attempt to create open communication to facilitate the flow of essential information. If the client interprets this as an invitation to be personal with the nurse, what are some techniques the nurse can use to set appropriate limits and continue the interview? (See Chapter 10 in your text for additional ideas.)

5. A client who gives a history of sexually transmitted disease should be asked specific questions related to that illness. List the minimum questions the nurse should ask on this subject.

6. Outline a symptom history for the client complaining of a self-discovered lump in the genital area.

7. In what way might substance abuse of any kind pose a direct threat to the male reproductive system?

8. During the history, questions about molestation are of great importance to a client of any age. What would be the advantage of asking such a question of a 20-year-old male? In what way might such a question be posed to a 6-year-old male?

9. Taking a drug history is important to the assessment of every body system. List some drugs that are known to have an impact on the male reproductive system.

10. Developmental assessment of the male reproductive system would include questions about both sexual and reproductive attitudes. What health promotion principles would you indicate as important to reproductive health?

11. The purpose of transilluminating the scrotum is to ensure the presence of _____ and to identify possible _____, _____, or _____.

12. External inspection of the perianal region could reveal several common problems. List at least three.

13. The rectal exam may be performed in the positions of client bending from the hips or side-lying. What is the advantage of the bending position if the client is capable?

14. In examination of the stool, how would the examiner discriminate from blood from a high gastrointestinal location and blood from an anal/rectal location?

REVIEW QUESTIONS

1. Gloves are used for examination of male genitalia to
   a. facilitate grasp of external organs.
   b. make masses easier to detect.
   c. prevent spread of unsuspected infection.
   d. protect the client from embarrassment.

2. The accepted definition of fertility is
   a. a sperm count of > 40,000.
   b. confirmation of ovulatory bleeding.

   c. history of a live birth.
   d. documentation of normal androgen levels.

3. Which of the following could impact sexual performance and/or fertility?
   a. so-called recreational drugs
   b. prescription drugs
   c. undescended testicle

d. emotional dysfunction
e. all of the above

4. When assessing the scrotum, the nurse should consider which of the following findings abnormal?
   a. The left testicle hangs slightly lower than the right, but both are equal in size.
   b. The scrotal skin has ridges (rugae) and is darker pigmented than the surrounding skin.
   c. Palpation reveals a small, smooth ropelike tissue felt through the posterolateral surface of the scrotum superior to the testes and ascending to the inguinal canal.
   d. There is darker hair on the scrotum.
   e. The scrotum is exquisitely tender to palpation.

5. Palpation of the testes should reveal
   a. equality of size.
   b. exquisite but brief tenderness.
   c. absence of testicular discharge.
   d. central placement.

6. A black tarry stool in an adult (melena) is a possible sign of
   a. jaundice.
   b. malabsorption.
   c. rectal bleeding.
   d. upper GI bleeding.

7. Inspection of the external genitalia focuses primarily upon skin and hair assessment.
   a. true
   b. false

8. If the client becomes uncomfortable during the focused interview related to rectal/genital/reproduction, end that phase of the interview and move on to more critical and less uncomfortable areas.
   a. good choice
   b. poor choice

9. The technique of palpation is not useful on the penis because the usual result of erection would interrupt the examination and invalidate any findings.
   a. true
   b. false

10. Your client tells you to be careful placing his suppository because he has rectal polyps that can be painful. What is your best response?
    a. Please be assured, I'll be gentle.
    b. Polyps should not be painful.
    c. Have you had these polyps evaluated by your doctor?

11. All of the following statements about hemorrhoids are true *except:* Hemorrhoids
    a. are dilated or varicosed veins.
    b. may be internal or external.

c. are always painful.
d. can become infected.
e. are discernible on inspection/palpation.

12. On routine exam, the prostate gland should be
    a. sensitive but nontender.
    b. free of excretion.
    c. asymmetrical.
    d. evaluated transurethrally.
    e. nonpalpable through the rectal mucosa.

13. Lack of central placement of the male urethra is no cause for concern as long as the tissue is normal and the client has no complaint.
    a. true
    b. false

14. On rectal examination, the examiner may assess (in whole or in part) the following: prostate gland, varicose veins, anal fissures, rectal mucosa, blood in the stool, and the tone of the rectal sphincters.
    a. true
    b. false

15. A complete assessment for hemorrhoids can be achieved by inspection of the perianal area.
    a. true
    b. false

16. Phimosis and paraphimosis are
    a. abnormal findings of the foreskin.
    b. the result of certain STDs.
    c. congenital variations of glans morphology.
    d. variations of cervical patency.

17. Scrotal swelling may be the result of
    a. generalized edema.
    b. hydrocele.
    c. indirect hernia.
    d. any of the above.

18. Cryptorchidism is a chronic form of orchitis.
    a. true
    b. false

19. Indirect inguinal hernia presents as
    a. eruption of testes into the internal inguinal ring.
    b. protrusion of abdominal contents into the inguinal canal or beyond.
    c. a mass felt abdominally in the inguinal area.
    d. often confused with inguinal lymphadenopathy.

20. Signs of syphilis that can be detected on physical exam include
    a. purulent discharge from the urethra.
    b. plaques on the dorsum of the penis.
    c. roughened skin with a wartlike appearance.

d. ulceration that is painless though reddened.

e. small vesicles on a reddened base.

21. Hydrocele differs from a scrotal hernia on physical assessment in that
    a. scrotal hernia is more painful.
    b. hydrocele will transilluminate.
    c. scrotal hernia is accompanied by history of inguinal hernia.
    d. hydrocele is a pediatric-only condition.

22. Orchitis differs from cancer of the testes on physical assessment in that
    a. orchitis is painful and often swollen.
    b. cancer of the testes is painful but never swollen.
    c. orchitis is accompanied by discharge.
    d. cancer is always accompanied by weight loss and lethargy.

23. The size of the testes does not change after puberty.
    a. true
    b. false

24. The primary concern with cryptorchidism is
    a. fertility.
    b. malignancy.
    c. testosterone levels.
    d. cosmetic.

25. Anal fissures are of concern because of the increased risk of
    a. rectal prolapse.
    b. hemorrhoids.
    c. infection.
    d. rectal polyps.

CASE STUDIES

1. David, 16 years of age, is in the primary care clinic for a sports checkup. In the course of history taking, the nurse asks him if he is sexually active. He tries to crack a few jokes and finally asks, "Who else is going to know what I say in here?" The nurse reassures him that his conversation will be confidential unless he gives information that indicates he has serious health needs. Then, he will be encouraged to share that information with whatever adults have responsibility for assisting him with his health needs. Thus reassured, David tells the nurse that he has been having sex with one girl, who was a virgin, so he doesn't have to "worry." Also, he thinks "she is probably too young at 15 years of age to get pregnant, and anyway I think she does something with pills."

   - What would you want to tell David about his actual risk of STD?

   - What would you want to tell him about the possibility of pregnancy?

   - What health promotion teaching would you do regarding specific protection against infection and his reproductive health in general?

   - What specific questions would you ask regarding the symptoms associated with the most common STDs?

   - What physical assessment procedures would you recommend for evaluation of David's reproductive system? Keep in mind that he is involved in sports on a regular basis.

   - Which nursing diagnoses could be applicable to David?

2. Henry is 36 years of age and is in the hospital for an inguinal hernia repair. It is the operative day and his course has been unremarkable. The nurse notes, however, that he began asking for his urinary catheter to be removed as soon as he awakened in the recovery room. The nurse reassures him that the catheter will be removed shortly but he continues to worry. The nurse asks him if the catheter is painful, which he denies. Finally he reveals that he is worried about a urinary infection because he has had some itching and burning in the recent past and thinks that the catheter may increase his chances of having a full-blown infection. The nurse admits that catheterization can

increase the risk of infection but that all safety precautions are taken and the procedure is a sterile one. Henry is clearly embarrassed and hastens to deny being unfaithful to his wife.

- What additional history would you need to evaluate the seriousness of Henry's symptoms? Outline a symptom history for possible urinary tract infection.

- What reassurance could you give Henry regarding his concern that you will think he has an STD?

- What physical signs can you look for on examination that may be associated with urinary tract infection?

- What health promotion teaching would you do regarding Henry's reproductive/renal health?

- Which nursing diagnoses could be applicable to Henry?

CLINICAL ACTIVITIES

Practicing with colleagues in asking sensitive questions is very helpful for preparing the beginning nurse to interact with the client in a professional manner. Practicing with laboratory models is equally helpful in readying the nurse for contact with a real client. Keep in mind that, almost invariably, models are stiffer and more difficult to position than are actual clients.

Practice taking a reproductive history with your lab partner, or with a client in the clinical area. Practice performing the physical assessment on available models, maintaining as formal an approach as you would with a client. Use the sample documentation form at the end of the chapter as a guideline.

- Protection from infection is crucial for both nurse and client in the actual assessment of the reproductive system.
- Gloves, clean drapes, towels, and any other equipment that will prevent spread of body fluids must be employed.

- Standard Precautions are of utmost importance in protecting the nurse and the client. Review these in Appendices B and C of your text.

It is essential that the examiner have an assistant/witness present during an assessment with an actual client.

- A relaxed yet formal approach to the client is helpful in maintaining maximum cooperation during the assessment.
- Should the "real client" become embarrassed during history or examination, it is usually helpful to acknowledge the obvious embarrassment with a supportive comment such as, "Your discomfort is very reasonable. We'll be finished shortly and discuss all of the findings."
- It is also important to ask the client if he has any questions both during and after the exam.
- For the male client, this is an opportune time to teach testicular self-examination and to suggest ways for the client to make this a routine part of his self-care.

Sample Documentation Form

Male Reproduction System

Name: _____ Date: _____

Age: _____ Gender: _____

Focused symptom analysis of current problem:

Reason for visit:

_____

Character: _____

Onset: _____

Duration: _____

Location: _____

Severity: _____

Associated problems: _____

Efforts to treat: _____

Current medications: _____

_____

History

Review of history related to male genitalia, hernia, and sexual function:

Children born: _____ Living: _____ Stepchildren: _____

YES/NO		If YES, provide details:

Genitals

☐	☐	History of problems	_____
☐	☐	STD	_____
☐	☐	Genital burning, itching	_____
☐	☐	Penis discharge	_____

Hernia

☐	☐	History of hernia (inguinal, scrotal)	_____
☐	☐	Bulge or fullness in inguinal area	_____
☐	☐	Groin-area pain or discomfort	_____

Urinary—Prostate

☐	☐	Kidney or urinary disease	_____
☐	☐	Frequent urination	_____
☐	☐	Difficult or painful urination	_____
☐	☐	Urinary incontinence	_____
☐	☐	Difficulty starting urination	_____
☐	☐	Dribbling following urination	_____
☐	☐	Feeling bladder not emptied	_____
☐	☐	Hematuria or foul-smelling urine	_____
☐	☐	Cancer history	_____

Scrotum

- ☐ ☐   Hernia   _____
- ☐ ☐   Swelling   _____
- ☐ ☐   Fertility   _____
- ☐ ☐   Testicular self-exam (Performs? Able to do?)   _____
- ☐ ☐   Lumps or lesions   _____

Sexual Function

- ☐ ☐   Sexually active   _____
- ☐ ☐   Number of partners   _____
- ☐ ☐   Gender of partners   _____
- ☐ ☐   Difficulty maintaining erection   _____
- ☐ ☐   Satisfied with performance   _____
- ☐ ☐   Sexual protection   _____
- ☐ ☐   Infertility problems   _____
- ☐ ☐   Family, life, job stress   _____
- ☐ ☐   Alcohol use   _____

Medical problems in other systems related to reproductive (diabetes, spinal cord injury, cardiovascular disease, neurologic disease, handicapping conditions): _____

_____

_____

Family history of problems of the reproductive system: _____

_____

_____

Physical Assessment

Protect the nurse with gloves and an assistant of the same sex as the client.

Inspection

General characteristics (genital skin color, swelling, redness, lesions, hair distribution, infestations, hygiene): _____

_____

_____

Penis (position, color, symmetry, contour, scars, venous pattern, pulsations, smegma, external meatus of urethra, urethral discharge): _____

_____

_____

Scrotum (skin color, symmetry, swelling, lesions, infestation; transilluminate if swollen):

_____

_____

Lymph (redness, swelling): _____

_____

_____

Palpation

Femoral arteries (pulse rate and quality, bilateral comparison): _____

_____

Inguinal lymph nodes (presence of lymph nodes, tenderness, enlargement, bilateral comparison):

_____

_____

Penis (tenderness, tissue consistency, retraction of foreskin, milk urethra—assess discharge):

_____

_____

Scrotum (testes bilateral, swelling, nodules, tenderness, masses): _____

Inguinal or femoral hernia (presence of hernia or bulge—bilateral assessment): _____

_____

See anus and rectum, below.

Analysis:

_____

_____

_____

_____

Anus, Rectum, and Prostate

History

Review of history related to anus, rectum, and prostate:

_____

YES/NO		If YES, provide details:

Stools

☐	☐	Change in bowel habits	_____
☐	☐	Difficulty with bowel movements	_____
☐	☐	Diarrhea	_____
☐	☐	Constipation	_____
☐	☐	Flatulence	_____
☐	☐	Fecal incontinence	_____
☐	☐	Routine use of laxatives	_____
☐	☐	Routine use of other bowel meds	_____

Stool characteristics

Frequency of bowel movements	_____
Color and consistency of stool	_____

Anus and Rectum

☐	☐	Anal or rectal bleeding	_____

Color of blood ☐ bright red ☐ black, tarry ☐ mixed

Associated with bowel movement ☐ yes ☐ no

☐	☐	Itching or pain	_____
☐	☐	Hemorrhoids	_____
☐	☐	Rectal polyps	_____
☐	☐	Colonoscopy	_____

Focused symptom analysis of current problem:

  Reason for visit:

_____

  Character: _____

  Onset: _____

  Duration: _____

  Location: _____

  Severity: _____

  Associated problems: _____

  Efforts to treat: _____

Physical Assessment

  Inspection

   Rectum (skin characteristics, hemorrhoids, lesions, skin tags, inflammation, drainage, prolapse):

_____

_____

_____

  Palpation

   Rectum (sphincter tone; internal or external hemorrhoids; rectal tone; presence of stool, pain, or tenderness; posterior rectal wall characteristics): _____

_____

   Drainage on glove after exam: _____

   Prostate (symmetry, consistency, mass, bulging into rectal wall, nodules, discomfort): _____

_____

_____

   Stool specimen for presence of occult blood: ☐ Positive

                                                     ☐ Negative

Analysis:

_____

_____

_____

_____

Nursing diagnoses: _____

_____

Female Reproductive System 22

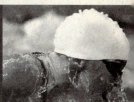

OVERVIEW

The female reproductive system is equally critical to maintenance of general health as it is to the specialized functions of reproduction and sexual pleasure. As with the male system, it is essential to life sustaining processes, such as tissue maintenance, absorption of critical elements and generation and maintenance of sexual characteristics. Problems in this system evidence themselves in biological, psychosocial, and psychological aspects of living. Additionally, culture plays a great role in client attitudes toward reproductive functioning and sexual mores. It is very important for the nurse to be sensitive to the values of both the nurse and the client in order to facilitate open and productive communication in providing care. By taking care to establish rapport and to initiate discussion in a comfortable and accepting manner, the nurse can elicit a more comprehensive and directive history than might have been otherwise possible. Techniques of examination must also be carried out in a manner consistent with client values and attitudes. A thorough history and physical examination provide the foundation for appropriate nursing diagnosis, treatment, and client education.

ASSIGNMENT

CD-ROM content: Chapter 22
Companion website: www.prenhall.com/damico, Chapter 22

VOCABULARY EXERCISE

After completing the reading assignment, you should be able to define the **key terms** listed below. Refer back to the page number from the main text for help.

Anteversion, 652
Antiflexion, 652
Bartholin's glands, 626
Cervical os, 628
Cervix, 628
Chadwick's sign, 629
Clitoris, 626
Cystocele, 643
Genital warts, 642
Goodell's sign, 629
Hymen, 643
Introitus, 626

Labia, 625
Ovaries, 628
Paraurethral glands, 626
Perineum, 643
Prolapsed uterus, 643
Rectocele, 643
Retroflexion, 652
Retroversion, 652
Uterine tubes, 628
Uterus, 628
Vagina, 626

ANATOMY EXERCISES

....

1. Label the external anatomical structures of the female reproductive system.

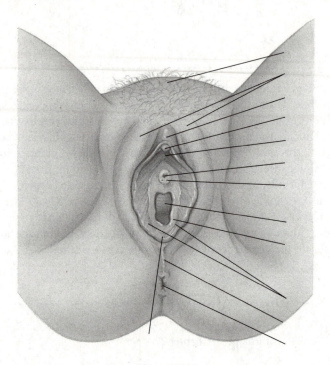

Figure 22–1

2. Note that all these structures are soft tissue structures, with skin and hair as major components. What are the clinical problems with skin and hair that could present in this genital area?

3. Referring to your response to question 2, what implications could these problems have for comfort?

4. Referring again to your response to question 2, what implications could these problems have for reproduction?

5. Label the internal anatomical structures of the female reproductive system.

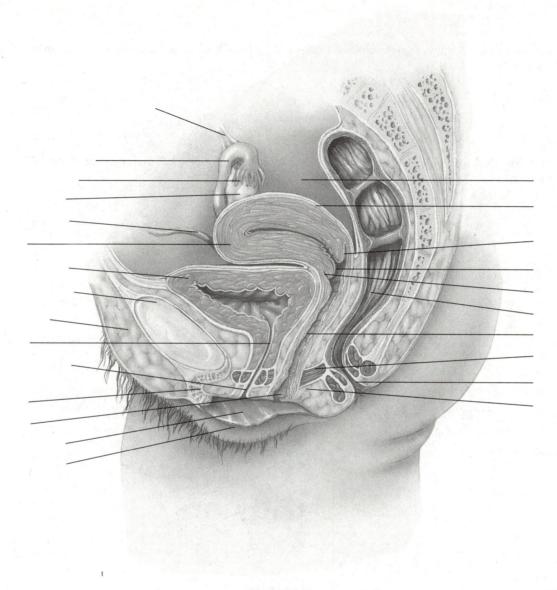

Figure 22–2

6. Note the nearness of the rectum to the vaginal canal. What effect might a full rectum have on the progress of labor?

7. Note the nearness of the uterus to the bladder. What effect might a full bladder have on the progress of labor?

8. Using Figure 22–2, draw arrows to indicate a change in the physiological uterus position to show anteversion and retroversion.

9. How does the length of the female urethra compare to the length of the male urethra? (See Chapter 21 for reference.) What clinical implications does this have?

10. Label the anatomical structures.

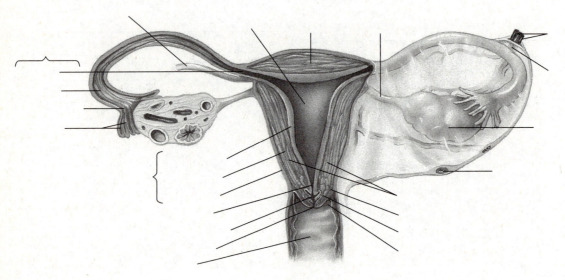

Figure 22–3

11. After labeling the structures indicated, trace the path of the egg from the ovary during ovulation. Then trace the path of ascending sperm through the vaginal canal up to the outer third of the fallopian tube. What impediments could interfere with the progress of either sperm or egg?

STUDY FOCUS

1. Interviewing for history of the reproductive system is enhanced by having a professional rapport with the client. What are the principles for the establishment of rapport with a client? Review Chapter 10 if necessary.

2. Many adolescents worry that they should be menstruating by age 12 or 13. If a young client is concerned that she is not yet menstruating at age 14, what can you tell her? What are the factors that influence menarche?

3. What are the general guidelines for considering a possibility of infertility? That is, for how long and at what frequency of sexual intercourse would it be considered that a client had given adequate exposure for pregnancy to occur?

4. One of the most common complaints of the reproductive system for the female is dysmenorrhea. Give a symptom outline for questions that would elicit complete information on a complaint of dysmenorrhea.

5. It is critical that the nurse ask about sexual orientation and sexual activity. What reassurances would encourage the client to be truthful and comprehensive?

6. The genital examination of a young child should only be done in the presence of the parent. What nursing intervention would contribute to the parent feeling at ease and able to ask pertinent questions?

7. Why is it important to ask the same focused interview questions of an older client as the nurse would ask of a younger woman?

8. During the inspection of genitalia, examination of genital hair yields two very important kinds of information. One is endocrine and one is integumentary. What are these features?

9. Speculum exam of the vagina is valuable in the assessment of mucous membrane and the appropriateness of reproductive structures. What features are important to evaluate in mucous membrane?

10. The bimanual exam is designed to evaluate position and tone. Discuss the expected finding on bimanual exam of a 20-year-old female who is sexually active but has never been pregnant.

11. A medication history is an important part of every system. Suggest at least two important questions for each of the following ages regarding medications the female client may be taking: an adolescent, a 30 year-old-female, and a 60-year-old female.

REVIEW QUESTIONS

1. Gloves are used for examination of female genitalia to
   a. facilitate grasp of external organs.
   b. make masses easier to detect.
   c. prevent spread of unsuspected infection.
   d. protect the client from embarrassment.

2. The accepted definition of fertility is
   a. a sperm count of > 40,000.
   b. confirmation of ovulatory bleeding.
   c. history of a live birth.
   d. documentation of normal hormonal levels.

3. Which of the following could impact sexual performance and/or fertility?
   a. so-called recreational drugs
   b. prescription drugs
   c. previous pelvic infection
   d. emotional dysfunction
   e. all of the above

4. The most important health history question for a female client is
   a. gravida, parity.
   b. last menstrual period.
   c. past medical or surgical gynecologic procedures.
   d. substance use or abuse.

5. Which is the proper technique for use of a speculum for vaginal examination?
   a. Press introitus downward; insert closed speculum obliquely or vertically.
   b. Spread labia; insert standard size speculum.
   c. Allow labia to spread; insert speculum slightly open.
   d. Insert one finger; insert opened speculum.

6. A black tarry stool in an adult (melena) is a possible sign of
   a. jaundice.
   b. malabsorption.
   c. rectal bleeding.
   d. upper GI bleeding.

7. In a nulliparous client, the cervical os normally looks
   a. X-shaped.
   b. round and closed.
   c. irregular.
   d. semicircular and slightly open.

8. Which of the following tests can best detect cervical cancer?
   a. Papanicolaou (Pap) test
   b. wet prep specimen
   c. vaginal pool specimen
   d. guaiac

9. A menstrual history is critical to assessment of the female
   a. of age 15 through 45.
   b. who is pregnant.
   c. of any age.
   d. who has been hysterectomized.

10. Inspection of the external genitalia focuses primarily upon skin and hair assessment.
    a. true
    b. false

11. If the client becomes uncomfortable during health history questioning related to rectal/genital/reproduction, end that phase of the interview and move on to more critical and less uncomfortable areas.
    a. good choice
    b. poor choice

12. Presence of vaginal discharge can be an indication of
    a. sexually transmitted disease.
    b. hormonal stimulation/endogenous or exogenous.
    c. sexual arousal.
    d. viral, bacterial, or fungal activity.
    e. any of the above.

13. Displacement of the uterus from midline position at any age, pregnant or nonpregnant, is
    a. an example of individual variation in the range of normal.
    b. an ominous sign of significant pathology.
    c. a finding that obligates the examiner to pursue etiology and discover cause.

Matching: Match the following self-care procedures with the recommendations that follow question 19.

14. Pap _____
15. mammogram (after 40 years of age) _____
16. breast self-exam _____
17. guaiac _____
18. urinalysis _____
19. analysis of discharge _____
    a. monthly basis
    b. only as needed
    c. yearly basis

20. Bluish coloration of vaginal mucosa can be a sign of
    a. bruising.
    b. progesterone influence.
    c. pregnancy.
    d. HPV infection.
    e. a, b, and c.

21. All of the following statements about hemorrhoids are true *except:* Hemorrhoids
    a. are dilated or varicosed veins.
    b. may be internal or external.
    c. are always painful.
    d. can become infected.
    e. are discernible on inspection/palpation.

22. On rectal examination, the examiner may assess in whole or in part (circle all that apply)
    a. the posterior aspect of the uterus.
    b. varicose veins.
    c. rectal polyps.
    d. rectal discharge.
    e. blood in the stool.
    f. tone of the rectal sphincters.

23. A complete assessment for hemorrhoids can be achieved by inspection of the perianal area.
    a. true
    b. false

24. Assessment of the Bartholin's glands would include
    a. palpation of the inguinal area.
    b. visual inspection of the rectovaginal wall.
    c. auscultation of the scrotum.
    d. bidigital palpation of the labia and vaginal wall.

25. Human papillomavirus, causative agent of venereal warts, is known conclusively to be associated with cancer of the cervix.
    a. true
    b. false

26. The **purpose** of the rectovaginal exam is to
    a. access the septum between the vagina and the rectum.
    b. obtain stool for guaiac testing.
    c. a and b.
    d. partially evaluate the uterus.
    e. a and d.

CASE STUDY

1. Carole is a 16-year-old high school student who has been sexually active for about 6 months. Upon discovering this, Carole's mother has insisted that she have a pelvic exam and a Pap smear. You are preparing Carole for her first exam and taking her history.

    - What specific questions would you ask about Carole's menses?

    - Why would you ask the age of her partner(s)?

    - What questions would you ask that would relate to signs of infection?

    When you begin to prepare Carole for her pelvic exam, she says, "My mother's just doing this to punish me. Why would the doctor go along with her? I think the whole idea is gross! I don't even know what is going to happen!" What can you tell Carole about the following:

    - why the doctor would agree to do this exam

    - exactly what to expect for the course of the exam

    - why this exam will be important for Carole now and in the future

    - questions that might be helpful to ask the doctor during or after the exam

    Which specific nursing diagnoses would apply to Carole at this point?

CLINICAL ACTIVITIES

Practicing with colleagues in asking sensitive questions is very helpful for preparing the beginning nurse to interact with the client in a professional manner. Practicing with laboratory models is equally helpful in readying the nurse for contact with a client. Keep in mind that, almost invariably, models are stiffer and more difficult to position than are actual clients.

Practice taking a reproductive history with your lab partner or with a client in the clinical area. Practice performing the physical assessment on available models, maintaining as formal an approach as you would with a client.

- Protection from infection is crucial for both nurse and client in the assessment of the reproductive system.
- Gloves, clean drapes, towels, and any other equipment that will prevent spread of body fluids must be employed.
- Review Standard Precautions in Appendices B and C of your text.

A relaxed yet formal approach to the client is helpful in maintaining maximum cooperation during the assessment.

- Should the "client" become embarrassed during history or examination, it is usually helpful to acknowledge the obvious embarrassment with a supportive comment such as, "Your discomfort is very reasonable. We'll be finished shortly and discuss all of the findings."

It is essential that the examiner have an assistant/witness present during an exam with an actual client.

- This is true regardless of the sex of the nurse and the client. This offers protection for both the client and the examiner.
- Use the guidelines and documentation forms at the end of this chapter to guide your practice.

Sample Documentation Form

Assessment of Female Reproductive System

Name: _____   Date: _____

Age: _____   Last Menstrual Period: _____

Gravida: _____   Parity: _____   AB: _____   Living Children: _____

Focused analysis of current problem:

    Reason for visit: _____

    _____

    Character: _____

    Onset: _____

    Duration: _____

    Location: _____

    Severity: _____

    Associated problems: _____

    Efforts to treat: _____

Current medications: _____

_____

History

Review of history related to female genitalia, gynecologic, and sexual function:

_____

YES/NO   If YES, provide details:

_____

Genitals and Gynecologic

☐	☐	History of surgery	_____
☐	☐	Reproductive concerns	_____
☐	☐	Gynecologic problems	_____
☐	☐	Hormonal therapy	_____
☐	☐	Genital burning, itching	_____
☐	☐	Vaginal burning, itching	_____
☐	☐	Vaginal, genitalia lesions	_____
☐	☐	Vaginal discharge problems	_____
☐	☐	Vaginal dryness	_____
☐	☐	Previous infections, STDs	_____
☐	☐	Pain and/or cramping problems	_____
☐	☐	Menopause symptoms	_____
☐	☐	Cancer history	_____

    Last Pap test   Date: _____

    Results: _____

    Menstrual history   Date of menarche: _____

    Date of last period: _____

    Regularity: _____

Flow characteristics: _____

Premenstrual symptoms: _____

Dysmenorrhea: _____

Usual treatment (dysmenorrheal): _____

Heavy/scanty bleeding: _____

Intermenstrual bleeding: _____

Hernia

☐ ☐   History of inguinal hernia   _____

☐ ☐   Bulge or fullness in inguinal area   _____

☐ ☐   Groin-area pain or discomfort   _____

☐ ☐   Femoral hernia   _____

☐ ☐   Umbilical hernia   _____

Urinary

☐ ☐   History urinary infections   _____

☐ ☐   Frequent urination   _____

☐ ☐   Difficult or painful urination   _____

☐ ☐   Malodorous urine   _____

☐ ☐   Urinary incontinence   _____

☐ ☐   Difficulty starting urination   _____

☐ ☐   Urgency feelings   _____

☐ ☐   Feeling bladder not emptied   _____

☐ ☐   Hematuria   _____

Sexual Function

☐ ☐   Sexual orientation   _____

☐ ☐   Sexually active   _____

☐ ☐   Satisfied with performance   _____

☐ ☐   Sexual protection   _____

☐ ☐   Fertility problems   _____

☐ ☐   Family, life, job stress   _____

☐ ☐   Substance use   _____

☐ ☐   Abuse experience   _____

Medical conditions affecting reproduction (diabetes, spinal cord injury, handicapping conditions): _____

_____

Lifestyle

Number of partners ☐ one partner   ☐ multiple partners

Partner gender   ☐ female ☐ male ☐ both

Obstetric History

☐ ☐   Pregnancies   _____

☐ ☐   Complications of pregnancy   _____

☐ ☐   Medical conditions affecting reproduction _____

☐ ☐   Fertility problems   _____

☐ ☐   Uses birth control (type)   _____

☐ ☐   Satisfied with birth control method _____

☐ ☐   Abuse during pregnancy   _____

Family history of genitalia, gynecologic, obstetric problems: _____

_____

_____

Physical Assessment

Inspection

General characteristics (genital skin color, swelling, redness, lesions, hair distribution, infestations, hygiene): _____

_____

External genitalia (color, symmetry, contour, scars, labia majora, labia minora, clitoris, urethral orifice, vaginal introitus, Skene's and Bartholin's glands, vaginal or urethral discharge): _____

_____

Perineum (scars, inflammation, lesions): _____

_____

Rectum (skin characteristics, hemorrhoids, lesions, skin tags, inflammation, drainage): _____

_____

Palpation

Labia (symmetry, consistency): _____

Perineum (competence, lesions, masses): _____

Introitus (size, shape, integrity, drainage): _____

Vaginal walls (competence, bulges, lesions, glands): _____

_____

Femoral arteries (pulse rate and quality, bilateral comparison): _____

_____

Inguinal lymph nodes (presence of lymph nodes, tenderness, enlargement, bilateral comparison):

_____

_____

Inguinal or femoral hernia (presence of hernia or bulge—bilateral assessment): _____

_____

Speculum Examination (Use Only Water as Lubricant)

General characteristics (vaginal wall color, lesions, nodules, moisture, exudate): _____

_____

Cervix (position, appearance, os, lesions, exudate): _____

_____

Specimens collected:
- ☐ Papanicolaou test: _____
- ☐ Gonococcal culture: _____
- ☐ Chlamydia swab: _____
- ☐ KOH wet mount for *Trichomonas*: _____
- ☐ Other: _____
- ☐ Other: _____

Bimanual Examination

Muscle tone (examiner's fingers in vagina—evaluate muscle tone as woman is instructed to squeeze pelvic muscles around examiner's fingers): _____

_____

Vaginal walls (tone, bulging): _____

_____

Uterus/cervix (position, size, shape, masses, tenderness, nodules, firmness, mobility): _____

_____

Adnexa and ovaries (ovary location, tenderness, size, consistency, nodules): _____

_____

Rectovaginal exam (tone of rectovaginal vault): _____

_____

Rectal examination

General characteristics (sphincter tone; hemorrhoids; presence of stool, pain, or tenderness; rectal wall consistency; polyps; posterior uterine wall characteristics): _____

_____

Stool specimen for presence of occult blood: ☐ Positive

                                                           ☐ Negative

Analysis:

_____

_____

Nursing diagnoses: _____

_____

Musculoskeletal System 23

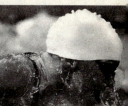

OVERVIEW

Assessment is very direct with the musculoskeletal system. Because its function is primarily motion and structure, much of the assessment can be done with very little enhancement, as the nurse observes the movement and support and assesses its competence. The system is, like all systems, very dependent on the proper functioning of the gastrointestinal system as it remodels itself constantly. If proper nutritional substrates are not consumed and absorbed, the system begins to fail.

In turn, proper functioning of the system provides for activity, exercise, the production of red blood cells, and the emergency storage of critical elements such as calcium. Failure in the system may be subtle, as with osteoporosis, or dramatic as with the trauma of fracture. Assessment, as with every system, is always based on symmetry and function.

ASSIGNMENT

CD-ROM content: Chapter 23, especially animations
Companion website: www.prenhall.com/damico, Chapter 23, especially Toolbox

VOCABULARY EXERCISE

After completing the reading assignment, you should be able to define the **key terms** listed below. Refer back to the page number from the main text for help.

Abduction, 674
Acetabulum, 670
Adduction, 674
Ballottement, 707
Bursae, 668
Calcaneus, 679
Circumduction, 674
Depression, 675
Dorsiflexion, 674
Elevation, 675
Eversion, 675
Extension, 674
Fibrous joint, 667
Flexion, 674
Fracture, 716
Gliding, 674
Hallux valgus, 723

Hyperextension, 674
Inversion, 675
Joint, 667
Kyphosis, 711
Lordosis, 711
Opposition, 675
Plantar flexion, 674
Pronation, 675
Protraction, 675
Retraction, 675
Rotation, 675
Scoliosis, 711
Subluxation, 681
Supination, 675
Synovial joint, 668
Tendon, 668
Tophi, 722

ANATOMY EXERCISES

1. Label the anatomical structures of the shoulder.

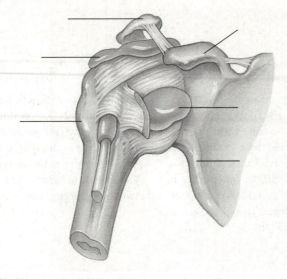

Figure 23–1

2. Look at the complexity of the shoulder joint. What is its natural range of motion?

3. Label the anatomical structures of the elbow.

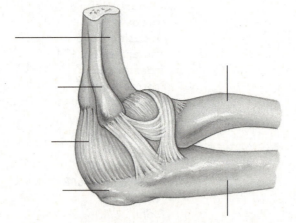

Figure 23–2

4. One of the most common complaints of the elbow is tendinitis. Looking at the joint and its intricate wrap of ligaments and tendons, what potential stresses would occur?

5. Label these anatomical structures of the hip.

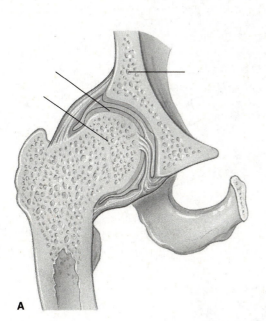

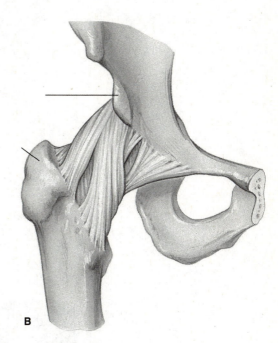

Figure 23–3

6. Looking at the hip in this figure, mark the area that you think would be most vulnerable to fracture.

7. Where might a prosthesis be placed?

8. Label the anatomical structures of the knee and great muscles.

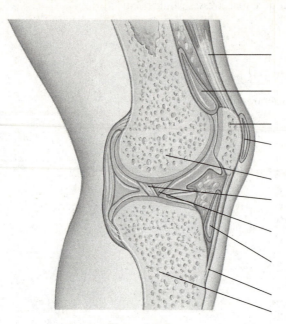

Figure 23–4

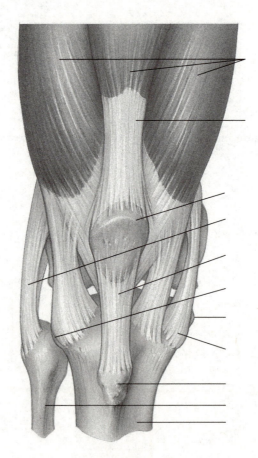

Figure 23–5

9. What are the main bones of the knee joint? What would you expect to be the result of a lateral blow to the knee?

STUDY FOCUS

1. How does the composition and structure of a bone reflect its range of expected performance? List the functions of bones as described in your text in Chapter 23, and relate those functions to the bone's structural components.

2. The passage of the fetus through the birth canal is a stressful one that may result in injuries to the infant. List the musculoskeletal injuries, and their presentations, that may occur during a vaginal birth (Chapters 25 and 26).

3. As aging advances, certain musculoskeletal changes are inevitable. Identify the changes discussed in your text, and the nursing actions that should be taken during the assessment of the musculoskeletal system of an older adult.

4. Outline a symptom history for complaint of pain or limited use of a limb by an adult client.

5. Many people self-treat discomforts of the musculoskeletal system. What are the common over-the-counter medications available? What are some alternative methods to relieve discomfort of muscles?

6. What health promotion advice would you give to a relatively sedentary person who expresses interest in beginning a sport for the purposes of improving fitness?

7. In every system, the general survey is an important assessment. In the musculoskeletal system, it is often the most useful component. List the aspects of the general survey that relate directly to the musculoskeletal system.

8. Each joint of the trunk and limb must be assessed for range of motion, strength, structure, symmetry, and shape. Describe the physical assessment for each joint.

9. Disorders of the musculoskeletal system fall into the categories of trauma, congenital defects, rheumatic defects, spinal abnormalities, and joint disorders. Does the nursing assessment differ among categories? If so, how?

REVIEW QUESTIONS

1. A goniometer is an instrument for testing the synovial membrane.
   a. true
   b. false

2. An audible and/or palpable crunching or grating of a joint is called
   a. fremitus.
   b. crepitation.
   c. rhonchi.
   d. friction rub.

3. Abnormal lateral curving of the thoracic spine is called
   a. lordosis.
   b. scoliosis.
   c. torticollis.
   d. kyphosis.

4. Abnormal exaggerated convexity of the thoracic spine is called
   a. lordosis.
   b. circumduction.
   c. ankylosis.
   d. kyphosis.

5. The range of motion of the knee includes flexion, extension, and which other type of movement?
   a. internal rotation
   b. circumduction
   c. inversion
   d. hyperextension
   e. none of the above

6. Normal range of motion for the hip includes flexion, extension, adduction, abduction, and which other type of movement?
   a. eversion
   b. pronation
   c. radial deviation
   d. rotation (internal and external)

7. When a client presents a history of musculoskeletal problems, the examiner should first examine affected body parts for reported problems.
    a. true
    b. false

8. The strength of the sternocleidomastoid muscle is evaluated by having the client
    a. clench his or her teeth during muscle palpation.
    b. extend his or her head against the examiner's hand.
    c. straighten his or her leg with examiner opposition.
    d. uncross his or her legs with examiner resistance.

9. Complete screening for scoliosis includes observing the client
    a. lying, sitting, and standing.
    b. standing and sitting.
    c. bending, twisting, and lifting.
    d. standing and bending.
    e. lying and twisting.

10. Which data from the health history could contribute to complaints of the musculoskeletal system?
    a. cigarette smoking, diet
    b. obesity
    c. competitive sports participation, sports conditioning
    d. immobility
    e. all of the above

11. Causes of abnormal gait include
    a. paralysis/partial paralysis and stress.
    b. muscle weakness and pain.
    c. joint injury/deterioration and lack of balance.
    d. fatigue and inequality of limbs.
    e. all of the above.

12. Mutable risk factors for osteoporosis include
    a. smoking and inadequate calcium.
    b. race, age, and gender.
    c. early-onset menopause.
    d. c and b.

13. If there is full range of motion on passive manipulation, limited range of motion on active manipulation could indicate
    a. paralysis.
    b. pain, inflammation, and infection.
    c. weakness.
    d. any or all of the above.

Matching: The nurse is assessing a client for resistance and muscle strength. Match the musculoskeletal test in the first column to the technique below question 17.

14. biceps _____

15. triceps _____

16. deltoids _____

17. quadriceps _____
    a. Client flexes leg at knee; nurse tries to extend knee.
    b. Client extends arms laterally, and nurse tries to push them down.
    c. Client tries to extend knee while nurse tries to flex knee.
    d. Client tries to flex arm into fighting position, and nurse tries to straighten forearm.
    e. Client tries to straighten or extend forearm while nurse tries to flex forearm.
    f. Client tries to cross arm across midline; nurse tries to prevent.

18. What dietary components are of greatest importance to the musculoskeletal system?

19. What drugs offer particular risks to the musculoskeletal system?

20. Cardinal signs of rheumatic disorders are _____, _____, _____, _____, and _____.

21. One abnormality of the spine is actually within normal limits for a toddler and a pregnant woman. This is
    a. scoliosis.
    b. lordosis.
    c. kyphosis.

22. Increased tone of an infant's muscles could signify
    a. an irritable baby.
    b. a period of anoxia.
    c. Dupuytren's contracture.

23. Osteoarthritis risk increases with (circle all that apply)
    a. repetitive motions.
    b. altered purine metabolism.
    c. age.
    d. muscle wasting conditions.
    e. obesity.

24. Rheumatoid arthritis characteristics include (circle all that apply)
   a. involvement of proximal joints of the hand.
   b. distal joint involvement.
   c. onset after 50 years of age.
   d. pain that improves with gentle use.
   e. pain that worsens with extended use.

25. When assessing strength in a muscle and joint, which factors beyond actual strength of the muscle may impact the findings?

CASE STUDIES

1. Charlie, a 14-year-old boy, presents with an injured leg in the school nurse's office, directly from the soccer field. He had kicked for a goal and then fell. He thinks he damaged his leg at about the ankle while kicking. Though there were other players involved in his fall, he does not think there was impact from anything other than the ball. After getting Charlie in a stable position, you start a history as you examine the injured leg.

   - What past medical history do you need?

   - What immediate lifestyle history do you need?

   - Outline a symptom history for the present problem.

   - What comorbid conditions would you worry about?

   As you examine the leg, you note a fairly enlarged ankle, no redness, and a normally shaped joint.

   - What comparison can you make to evaluate the size of the ankle?

   - How would you assess pain? (Review Chapter 8 for helpful suggestions.)

   - Would you use active or passive range of motion for assessment of the ankle at this point?

   - When Charlie is recovered from this injury, what health promotion teaching might you attempt for this young soccer player?

   - What nursing diagnoses might apply?

2. Imelda, a 30-year-old secretary, presents at a primary care clinic with complaints of a sore back. She denies lifting heavy objects, or impact injuries. She states she does not spend long amounts of time on her feet. As a matter of fact, she states, she spends her entire workday sitting at a desk. Other than necessary shopping and the preparation of a meal for herself and her husband, her hobbies and recreation are all sedentary. Imelda admits to being overweight and says that she avoids dairy products because they are so fattening. She has been taking aspirin and ibuprofen for her back but thinks she may need something stronger.

   - What family history may be important?

   - In a medication history, what drugs would be of concern to her musculoskeletal system?

   - In a dietary history, what factors are of major importance?

   - What would be red flags in a past medical history?

   - What additional information do you need about the aspirin and ibuprofen?

   - Why is it important to take a complete pain history?

On physical assessment:

- What would your first assessment be?

- In assessment of the spine, what range of motion would you expect? What spinal curves would you expect?

- Where would you assess sensation?

Follow-up health teaching:

- What health promotion teaching would you do once it is confirmed that Imelda is well enough to sustain normal activity?

- What dietary teaching might be appropriate?

- What nursing diagnoses apply to Imelda?

CLINICAL ACTIVITIES

Plan to do this part of a complete assessment when the client will not be too tired to perform at his or her best.

- If the client has a painful chronic condition, plan pain relief so that the client can perform without increasing discomfort.
- Assessment of the musculoskeletal system is very direct. Findings are also apparent to the client, so encouragement and support are quite important. It will be clear to the client when he or she cannot complete a request for movement or strength, and this may be distressing. Be supportive and move on to the next part of the assessment without undue focus on a failed part.

- Remember that normal and average are two different things. It is actually normal for an adult person to be able to run for 5 miles. It is probably not average. More so than other systems, the musculoskeletal exam varies greatly with developmental levels in terms of strength and range of motion.
- Complete a musculoskeletal history and then physical assessment on your lab partner or client. Use the comprehensive information in your text and the sample documentation form at the end of the chapter as a guideline.

Sample Documentation Form

Musculoskeletal Assessment

Name: _____ Date: _____

Age: _____ Gender: _____

History

Review of history related to musculoskeletal system:

_____

YES/NO   If YES, provide details:

_____

Musculoskeletal

☐	☐	Musculoskeletal disease	_____
☐	☐	Recent injury	_____
☐	☐	Exercise history	_____
☐	☐	Muscle aches or pain	_____
☐	☐	Skeletal aches or pain	_____
☐	☐	Muscle weakness or limitation	_____
☐	☐	Joint pain or stiffness	_____
☐	☐	Muscular disease/disorder	_____
☐	☐	Neck pain/problem	_____
☐	☐	Back pain/problem	_____
☐	☐	Shoulder pain/problem	_____
☐	☐	Elbow pain/problem	_____
☐	☐	Hand or wrist pain/problem	_____
☐	☐	Hip pain/problem	_____
☐	☐	Knee pain/problem	_____
☐	☐	Ankle pain/problem	_____
☐	☐	Foot pain/problem	_____
☐	☐	Fracture history	_____
☐	☐	Change in gait or mobility	_____
☐	☐	Musculoskeletal surgery	_____
☐	☐	Dietary calcium, protein intake	_____
☐	☐	Chronic disease	_____
☐	☐	Bone density evaluation	_____

Current medications: _____

_____

Allergies: _____

_____

Family history/musculoskeletal system: _____

_____

Review of history related to the current visit:

  Focused symptom analysis of current problem:

   Reason for visit: _____

   _____

   Character: _____

   Onset: _____

   Duration: _____

   Location: _____

   Severity: _____

   Associated problems: _____

   Efforts to treat: _____

Physical Assessment:

  Inspection

   General survey (posture, body symmetry, gait, deformities, skeletal development, muscle development): _____

   _____

   _____

   _____

  Inspection/Palpation

   Spine (cervical, thoracic, lumbar, sacral curvatures; tenderness; redness; swelling; deformities):

   _____

   _____

   Active and passive ROM (flexion, extension, rotation, lateral bending; pain limitation): _____

   _____

   _____

   Shoulders, elbows (contour, deformity, tenderness, redness, swelling, crepitus): _____

   _____

   _____

   Shoulders, active and passive ROM (shoulder internal/external rotation, flexion, extension, pain, limitation): _____

   _____

   Elbow (flexion, extension, pronation, supination, pain limitation): _____

   _____

   _____

   Wrists, fingers (size, shape, symmetry, contour, redness, swelling, deformity, tenderness, crepitus):

   _____

   _____

   Forearm, active and passive ROM (flexion, extension, hyperextension, circumduction, radial/ulnar deviation; pain limitation): _____

   _____

Hips and knees (contour, size, symmetry, redness, swelling, deformity, tenderness, crepitus):

_____

_____

Hips, active and passive ROM (internal/external rotation, flexion, extension; pain, limitation): _____

_____

_____

Knees (flexion, extension, hyperextension; pain, limitation): _____

_____

_____

Ballottement: _____

Ankles, toes (size, shape, symmetry, deformities, redness, tenderness, swelling): _____

_____

Ankles and feet, active and passive ROM (flexion, extension, hyperextension, inversion, eversion; pain, limitation): _____

_____

Muscle Stength

Muscle strength evaluation (bilateral evaluation and comparison of all muscle groups by testing extension and flexion of the muscle groups against resistance): _____

_____

_____

Functional Assessment

Walking distance: _____

Climbing stairs: _____

Dressing/grooming: _____

Rise from chair: _____

Rise from bed: _____

Toileting/bathing: _____

Analysis:

_____

_____

_____

_____

_____

Nursing diagnoses: _____

_____

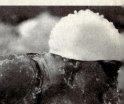

OVERVIEW

The neurologic system is the great command and communications center. Though enormously complex, the system can be assessed very directly. Reasons for impaired system responses may be complex and difficult to diagnose, but the assessment can be done by a skilled nurse with a careful and sensitive approach to the client.

While much of the neurologic system is objectively performance oriented, cognitive and affective functions are heavily dependent on education, culture, and language. For example, if a client doesn't recognize an object because it is outside his cultural experience, it is difficult to analyze his response as neurologic versus cultural. If he can't remember certain orientation data because he is highly anxious, does he have an orientation problem or an anxiety problem? Therefore, great care must be taken by the nurse to prepare the client and to understand impediments that may inhibit successful responses during testing.

ASSIGNMENT

CD-ROM content: Chapter 24, especially animations
Companion website: www.prenhall.com/damico, Chapter 24, especially Toolbox

VOCABULARY EXERCISE

After completing the reading assignment, you should be able to define the **key terms** listed below. Refer back to the page number from the main text for help.

Analgesia, 762
Anesthesia, 762
Anosmia, 747
Babinski response, 771
Brain stem, 732
Central nervous system, 731
Cerebellum, 732
Cerebrum, 732
Clonus, 767
Coma, 773
Dermatome, 733
Diplopia, 748
Dysphagia, 753
Hypalgesia, 762

Hyperesthesia, 762
Meninges, 731
Nuchal rigidity, 772
Nystagmus, 748
Papilledema, 748
Peripheral nervous system, 731
Reflexes, 733
Retrobulbar neuritis, 748
Romberg's test, 758
Seizures, 775
Spinal cord, 732
Syncope, 773
Thalamus, 732

ANATOMY EXERCISES

1. The lobes of this figure of the brain are labeled. Next to each lobe, note the activity for which each lobe is responsible.

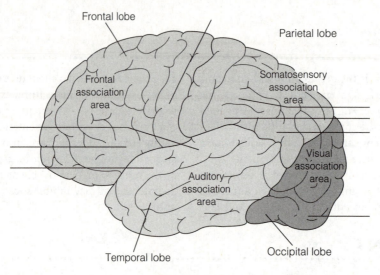

Figure 24–1

2. If an injury, such as a stroke or an aneurysm, should occur to the parietal lobe, what functions would be disturbed?

3. If an injury, such as a stroke or an aneurysm, should occur to the temporal lobe, what functions would be disturbed?

4. If an injury, such as a stroke or an aneurysm, should occur to the occipital lobe, what functions would be disturbed?

5. Label the groups of spinal nerves.

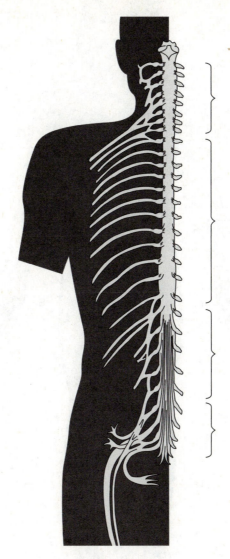

Figure 24–2

6. If an injury should occur to the cervical spinal nerves, what symptoms would be presented?

7. Are spinal nerves motor or sensory?

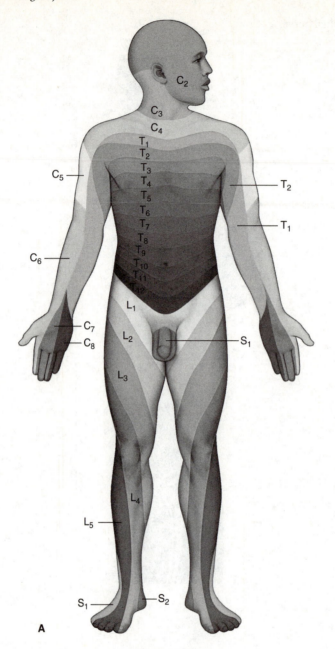

A

Figure 24–3a

8. Follow the distribution of the pairs of spinal nerves. What are the shaded distributions called? Of what help are they to the nurse who is assessing a client?

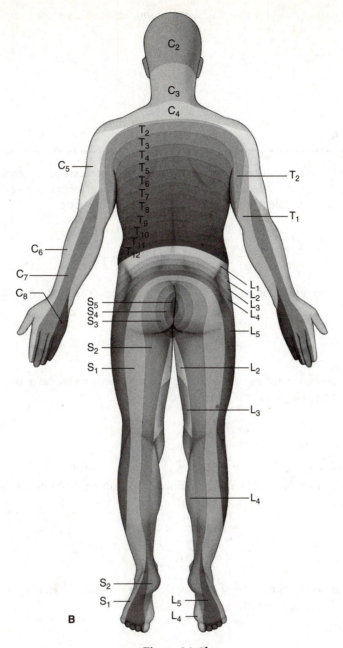

Figure 24–3b

9. If a client complained of pain in the knee and the knee was normal to evaluation, what might be an additional possibility?

10. Where would a client with a herpes zoster infection of T_6 see an eruption of herpes rash?

11. A client with numbness detected in the sole of the left foot should be evaluated for compression or injury of which spinal nerve?

STUDY FOCUS

1. Reflexes are the basic defense structures of the human body. What reflexes are present in all ages? What special reflexes are present in the neonate and infant that disappear as the infant gains some self-protective skills? Do adult reflexes disappear in the healthy older adult? What changes occur with aging?

2. Describe the types and importance of language barriers that may affect assessment of the neurologic system.

3. Changes in ability to carry out activities of daily living may have a neurologic basis. If a client complains of a lack of secure balance, what neurologic structure could be involved?

4. Clients may use terms such as light-headedness, dizziness, and fainting. As a nurse, how would you differentiate between these terms?

5. Substance abuse can present with neurologic deficits. Describe a focused history the nurse would take if a client admitted to the abuse of a drug, or drugs.

6. What dietary implications exist for the neurologic system?

7. The Mini-Mental State Exam is frequently used in general practice. What are its major components? What are its limitations?

8. In testing any aspect of the neurologic system, the nurse must be sure the client understands the instructions for performance. What is a good way of assessing that the client understands?

9. What are the primary features of a reflex?

10. List health promotion concerns relative to the neurologic system for the child, the adult, and the elderly.

REVIEW QUESTIONS

1. Your client reports an increased frequency of falls or accidents. This can be a sign of
   a. neurologic deficit (sensation, coordination, etc.).
   b. fatigue.
   c. stress/anxiety.
   d. muscle weakness.
   e. any of the above.

2. Your client complains of sudden onset of high fever accompanied by headache and "stiff neck." He tells you he had meningitis last year. At this time, meningitis would be considered
   a. certain diagnosis.
   b. past medical history.
   c. an unnecessary worry.
   d. very unlikely to strike twice.

3. Nuchal rigidity refers to
   a. rigid thought patterns.
   b. nuchal cord compression.
   c. pain and resistance to neck flexion.

4. The 12 pairs of cranial nerves supply all of the following areas **except**
   a. the head.
   b. the heart.
   c. the neck.
   d. the brain.

5. A reflex is a defense mechanism of the nervous system that operates consciously.
   a. true
   b. false

6. The trigeminal nerve (cranial nerve V) affects the muscles of mastication and the sensation of taste.
   a. true
   b. false

7. Which of the following is the most often used technique for assessment of the neurologic system?
   a. inspection
   b. palpation
   c. percussion
   d. auscultation

8. Signs and symptoms that should alert the examiner to possible neurologic dysfunction include
   a. decreased hearing ability and difficulty speaking clearly.
   b. dilated pupils in bright light.
   c. disequilibrium.
   d. loss of temperature sense.
   e. any of the above.

9. Which of the following would not test proprioception and coordination?
   a. Close eyes and touch nose with finger.
   b. Hop on first one foot and then the other.
   c. Run heel of foot up and down opposite shin.
   d. Distinguish between sharp and dull sensation.
   e. a, b, and c

10. A client with physiological sensation would be better able to discriminate two point sensation in which of the following structures?
    a. conjunctiva
    b. trunk
    c. fingertips
    d. upper arms

11. Which of the following is a valid and reliable tool for assessing neurologic status of a client with altered consciousness?
    a. Kernig's tool
    b. Glasgow Coma Scale
    c. Serial 7's

12. Which of the following would not be a reason for lack of muscle group symmetry (right side to left side)?
    a. neurologic impairment
    b. musculoskeletal impairment
    c. nutritional disorder
    d. significant overuse of one side
    e. none of the above

13. When is the mental status portion of the neurologic system examination performed?
    a. during the history-taking process
    b. during assessment of cranial nerves and deep tendon reflexes
    c. during the time when questions related to memory are asked
    d. constantly, throughout the entire interaction with a client

14. Evaluation of mental status requires the examiner to have basic knowledge of the client's
    a. neurologic status.
    b. culture.
    c. level of intelligence and education.
    d. all of the above.

15. Appropriateness of emotional affect can be evaluated by
    a. cranial nerve testing.
    b. communication.
    c. visual inspection.
    d. evaluation of muscle strength.
    e. b and c.

16. You may ask the client to follow a series of short reasonable commands to assess
    a. judgment.
    b. attention span.
    c. arithmetic calculations.
    d. abstract reasoning.

17. You notice that your client's right eyelid droops, though the left lid is appropriate. Your client may
    a. be sleepy.
    b. have dysfunction of cranial nerve V (trigeminal).
    c. have dysfunction of cranial nerve VII (facial).
    d. have unilateral exophthalmos.

18. The features of a seizure that are most helpful to identify to assist in appropriate treatment are _____, _____, and _____.

19. Identify three chronic diseases that increase the risk of neurologic impairment.

20. Inability to discriminate between two or three familiar scents is called
    a. anisocoria.
    b. anosmia.
    c. cranial nerve II dysfunction.
    d. hypalgesia.

21. The ability to identify a familiar object through blind touch is called
    a. stereognosis.
    b. graphesthesia.
    c. proprioception.
    d. ataxia.

22. A walk characterized by spastic limbs and a stiff jerky movement is called
    a. festination gait.
    b. ataxic gait.
    c. scissors gait.
    d. steppage gait.

23. A continual rapid short spasm involving a muscle or muscle group is called
    a. dystonia.
    b. myoclonus.
    c. athetoid movement.
    d. a tic.

24. Health promotion questions relative to head trauma should include inquiries about (circle all that apply)
    a. seat belt use.
    b. substance abuse.
    c. protective head gear for hobbies.
    d. protective head gear for work activities.
    e. child car seat use and safety.

25. List the risk factors for stroke.

CASE STUDY

You see Tom Bradley on the morning of his scheduled surgery for hernia. He is a 28-year-old retail worker in apparent good health except for the inguinal hernia, which has been aggravated by lifting. He was admitted the previous day for routine lab work and has been in the hospital for about 16 hours. As you take his preoperative history, you note that he mentions various sports that he "used to play" but no longer finds the time. He admits to frequent headaches and states that he has one today. As you do a general survey, you are surprised to note a fine tremor in his hands. As he gets up to go to the bathroom, you observe a somewhat unsteady gait.

- What focused health history questions need to be asked relative to the change in lifestyle, tremor, and unsteady gait?

- What aspects of the personal social history may be especially relevant?

- Is it appropriate to call attention to the observable tremor?

- How could you phrase questions about the unsteady gait?

- What specific neurologic exams would you perform to have objective findings regarding the tremor and gait?

- Though such movement disorders as Parkinson's disease are possible in a 28-year-old, what are some other possibilities?

- What additional assessments could you do to rule in or rule out these diagnoses?

- What nursing diagnoses might apply to Mr. Bradley?

CLINICAL ACTIVITIES

Prepare to take a history and to perform a complete neurologic exam on a client or on your lab partner or willing volunteer.

▶ In taking the history, allow time and direction to gain a knowledge of the client's ability to perform activities of daily living and to describe any changes that he or she has noted in competence.

▶ In performing the physical assessment, take care to give clear and complete instructions to your client and to use objects and language that are familiar to the client.

▶ If there is any possibility of your client losing balance, be sure to have protection and help available. Note that it is almost impossible to catch a falling adult, even a very small person.

Use the sample documentation form at the end of the chapter as a guideline to assist you in a complete assessment and a comprehensive documentation.

Sample Documentation Form

Neurologic Assessment

Name: _____ Date: _____

Age: _____ Gender: _____

History

Review of history related to neurologic system:

_____

YES/NO   If YES, provide details:

_____

General Neurologic

☐ ☐ Mental illness _____

☐ ☐ Neurologic disease _____

☐ ☐ Severe or persistent headaches _____

☐ ☐ Head injury _____

☐ ☐ Convulsions _____

☐ ☐ Tremor/weakness _____

☐ ☐ Recent injury _____

☐ ☐ Speech difficulty _____

☐ ☐ Numbness/tingling _____

☐ ☐ Neurologic pain _____

☐ ☐ Dysphagia _____

☐ ☐ Gait problems _____

☐ ☐ Coordination problems _____

☐ ☐ Dizziness _____

☐ ☐ Spinal cord injury _____

☐ ☐ Memory difficulties _____

☐ ☐ Learning disorder _____

☐ ☐ Substance abuse _____

Sleep pattern/difficulties: _____

_____

Allergies (and responses): _____

_____

_____

Current medications: _____

_____

Family history of problems relating to the neurologic system: _____

_____

Review of history related to the current visit:

   Focused symptom analysis of current problem:

      Reason for visit: _____

_____

      Character: _____

      Onset: _____

      Duration: _____

      Location: _____

      Severity: _____

      Associated problems: _____

      Efforts to treat: _____

Physical Assessment

   Mental Status

      LOC (level of consciousness): _____

      Orientation (person, time, place): _____

      Dress and grooming: _____

      Behavior (appropriateness): _____

      Speech (intelligible, pace): _____

      Mood/affect (facial expression, attitude): _____

      Memory (recent, remote): _____

      Cognitive (reading, writing, abstract reasoning, judgment): _____

      Thought processes (content, logic): _____

      Suicidal thoughts (spontaneous expression, response to examiner): _____

_____

      See also Mini-Mental State Examination

   Inspection

      General characteristics (posture, body position, noted weaknesses, tremor): _____

_____

_____

Cranial Nerves

	CRANIAL NERVE	ASSESSMENT	FINDINGS
I	Olfactory	• Smell • Odor recognition	
II	Optic	• Visual acuity • Visual fields	
III	Oculomotor	• Raise eyelids • Extraocular eye movements	
IV	Trochlear	• Eye movement—inward and downward	
V	Trigeminal	• Chewing • Clenching teeth • Sensations to the face	
VI	Abducens	• Lateral eye movements	
VII	Facial	• Facial expressions • Taste—anterior two-thirds of tongue • Secretion tears and saliva	
VIII	Acoustic	• Hearing • Equilibrium	
IX	Glossopharyngeal	• Swallowing • Gag reflex • Taste—posterior third of tongue • Salivary gland secretion	
X	Vagus	• Speech phonation • Swallowing • Sensation behind ear • Gag reflex	
XI	Spinal Accessory	• Turn head • Shrug shoulders	
XII	Hypoglossal	• Tongue movement	

Motor Function

General characteristics (general response, client cooperation):

_____

_____

Place check in □ of technique used. Record appropriate findings.

MOTOR FUNCTION	TECHNIQUE USED	Findings: Tone, Strength
Gross Motor	□ Ambulation	
	□ Gait	
Proprioception and Cerebellar Function **Balance**	□ Romberg	
Proprioception and Cerebellar Function	□ Finger-to-finger touching	
Fine Motor—Upper Extremities	□ Rapid alternating movements	
Proprioception and Cerebellar Function	□ Heel-to-shin movement	
Fine Motor—Lower Extremities	□ Heel-toe walking	

Sensory Function

General characteristics (general response, client cooperation): _____

_____

_____

Place check in □ of technique used. Record appropriate findings.

SENSORY FUNCTION	TECHNIQUE USED	FINDINGS
Touch	□ Superficial touch sensation	
	□ Temperature sensation	
	□ Sensation of position	
	□ Pressure sensation	
	□ Vibratory sensation over bony prominence	
	□ Two-point discrimination	
	□ Alternating sharp dull	
Cortical Sensory	□ Correct identification of object (stereognosis)	
	□ Two-point discrimination	
	□ Correct identification of marking (graphesthesia)	

Deep Tendon Reflexes

General characteristics (body position, tendon response, client cooperation): _____

_____

_____

TENDON REFLEX	ASSESSMENT	REPORTED GRADE	
Biceps Tendon	Biceps contraction and forearm flexion at the elbow	Right	
		Left	
Triceps Tendon	Contraction of the triceps muscles with extension of the elbow	Right	
		Left	
Brachioradialis Tendon	Forearm supination with flexion at the elbow	Right	
		Left	
Patellar Tendon	Contraction of the quadriceps muscle with knee extension	Right	
		Left	
Achilles Tendon	Plantar flexion of the foot	Right	
		Left	
Plantar Tendon (Babinski)	Flexion of toes inward and downward	Right	
		Left	
REFLEX GRADE	++++	Brisk, hyperactive, clonus of tendon	
	+++	More brisk than expected	
	++	Normal	
	+	Slightly diminished response	
	0	No response	

Analysis:

_____

_____

_____

Nursing diagnoses: _____

_____

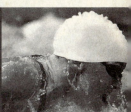

25

OVERVIEW

From infant to adolescent is a huge range of variation in biology and life tasks. Much of the previously presented content of this book is appropriate to this age range with minor modification, but some additional content is necessary as well. The developmental profile can change drastically in very short periods of time. Focused interview questions, health promotion concerns, and risk factors must be age related. Equally important is the approach to the client in terms of rapport and of promoting cooperation. With infants and children, rapport is important. The physical assessment must be planned to allow for client cooperation. Privacy is a high priority when dealing with adolescents.

ASSIGNMENT

CD-ROM content: Chapter 25, especially clinical spotlight videos
Companion website: www.prenhall.com/damico, Chapter 25

VOCABULARY EXERCISE

After completing the reading assignment, you should be able to define the **key terms** listed below. Refer back to the page number from the main text for help.

Acrocyanosis, 786
Adolescence, 783
Anterior fontanel, 786
Atopic dermatitis, 786
Caput succedaneum, 787
Cephalocaudal, 783
Cephalohematoma, 787
Choanal atresia, 790
Coarctation of the aorta, 790
Cranial sutures, 787
Craniosynostosis, 787
Cryptorchidism, 792
Ductus arteriosus, 790
Ductus venosus, 790
Eczema, 786
Epiphyseal plates, 792
Foramen ovale, 790
Genu valgum, 792
Genu varum, 792
Gynecomastia, 791
Infant, 783
Innocent murmur, 790
Labial adhesion, 792
Lambdoidal sutures, 787

Lanugo, 786
Laryngomalacia, 790
Macrocephaly, 802
Metopic sutures, 787
Microcephaly, 802
Milia, 786
Mongolian spots, 786
Morbilliform, 786
Muscular dystrophy, 792
Newborns, 783
Otitis media, 787
Posterior fontanel, 786
Preschooler, 783
Sagittal suture, 787
Salmon patches, 786
School age, 783
Scoliosis, 792
Sinus arrhythmia, 790
Teratogens, 797
Thelarche, 791
Toddler, 783
Tracheomalacia, 790
Umbilical hernia, 792
Vernix caseosa, 786

ANATOMY EXERCISES

The Newborn's Head

1. Label the cranial sutures and fontanelles drawn on the newborn's head.

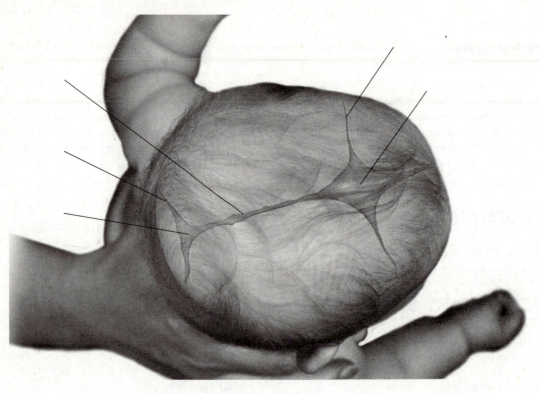

Figure 25–1

2. What is the purpose of the immature cranial sutures for the infant and mother?

3. Of what use are these landmarks to healthcare providers during prenatal and intrapartal assessment?

4. Of what importance are these landmarks in the ongoing assessment of the infant and toddler?

STUDY FOCUS

1. As important as nutrition is to every age, it is doubly critical in assessment of the developing infant, toddler, preschooler, and adolescent. List the major nutrition risks for the following ages.

   Newborn:

   Infant:

Toddler:

Preschooler:

School-age child:

Adolescent:

2. Clinical evaluation of nutrition includes assessment of skin, hair, nails, skeleton, and the endocrine system. Discuss the problems of under- and overnutrition in the given age categories.

3. The skin of the newborn and infant is a maze of lesions not seen in adulthood. Most of these variations are benign and resolve by toddler age. List and briefly describe these lesions.

4. Vital signs are significantly different in the newborn, infant, and toddler. Give the expected range of normal for vital signs for newborns, infants, toddlers, and school age children.

5. Transition from the fetal to the extrauterine stage of life includes major pulmonary and cardiovascular shifts. What are these transitions, and how long does the infant have to accomplish this shift?

6. Genitourinary evaluation is important at each well-child exam. What developmental milestone is related to each of the following?

Bladder capacity:

Appropriateness of genitalia:

Eruption of secondary sex characteristics:

7. Certain reflexes in children assert and then resolve when no longer needed. What functions do the following reflexes have?

Rooting:

Palmar grasp:

Stepping:

8. Adolescents are experiencing and questioning physical and emotional changes at the same time they are seeking privacy and control. What specific efforts can the nurse make to address these needs?

9. Very young children are especially vulnerable to eye, nose, and throat infections. What is the anatomical and biological basis for this vulnerability?

10. Eye assessments in children are very important because growth directly affects the shape of the eyeball and its rectus muscles. Discuss features of an eye assessment for the following ages.

    Newborn/infant:

    Toddler:

    Preschooler:

    Adolescent:

11. In which systems should the possibility of abuse be considered in evaluating findings?

REVIEW QUESTIONS

1. Acrocyanosis is defined as
    a. a blotchy, hivelike rash found on a newborn.
    b. a nonelevated purplish birthmark at the base of the spine.
    c. transient bluish discoloration of an infant's hands and feet on exposure to cold.
    d. plugged sebaceous glands.

2. In the newborn, it is usually possible to palpate how many fontanels?
    a. two
    b. four
    c. six
    d. eight

3. How should the nurse elicit the Moro reflex in a neonate?
    a. Apply pressure to the base of the toes.
    b. Touch the cheek.
    c. Allow a properly supported infant in a semi-sitting position to drop back to a 30-degree angle.
    d. b and c.

4. A pulse rate of 160 in a baby who had just been crying would probably indicate
    a. normalcy.
    b. infection.
    c. heart disease.
    d. respiratory distress syndrome.

5. An area of swelling of the newborn's scalp that exactly follows the contour of the skull sutures could be a
    a. caput succedaneum.
    b. cephalohematoma.
    c. molding.
    d. craniotabes.

6. Information on the newborn infant's personal/social/family history should, if possible, include
    a. age of parents, number of siblings, and ethnic culture of expected primary caregivers (parents, guardians, etc.).
    b. maternal fetal blood incompatibility and maternal substance exposures during gestation.
    c. knowledge of parents/guardians of child rearing.
    d. all of the above.

7. Types of maternal exposures of concern relative to a newborn infant include
    a. chemical.
    b. microorganic.
    c. severe or continuous stress.
    d. nutritional.
    e. all of the above.

8. An exposed term newborn with dusky bluish discoloration over the sacrum and bluish discoloration of hands and feet is likely (based on this data alone)
    a. in cardiovascular compromise.
    b. in respiratory compromise.
    c. a normal newborn.
    d. a preterm infant.

9. A normal newborn is expected to have an irregular
    a. respiratory pattern.
    b. cardiac pattern.
    c. none of the above.

10. Assessing descent of testes in the newborn male and presence of vaginal orifice in the newborn female are examples of
    a. exams that can be delayed to 1 year of age.
    b. sexual abuse of an infant.
    c. assessing reproductive development.

True or False: Use the letter "a" if the answer is true. Use the letter "b" if the answer is false.

11. Slow head growth of a child would be much less serious than rapid head growth. _____

12. Physiologic jaundice in newborns appears within the first 24 hours. _____

13. Mongolian spots are seen more often in the brown and black races and have no clinical significance. _____

14. A respiratory rate of 50/min in a newborn is significantly above normal. _____

15. On abdominal exam, hernia would be an unlikely finding in a newborn. _____

16. An ophthalmic exam of the newborn is crucial, but it requires only determination of the red light reflex and pupillary response. _____

17. All upper and lower deciduous teeth are in place by
    a. 6 months.
    b. 7 years.
    c. 2½ years.
    d. 18 months.

18. A finding of cyanosis in a toddler is more likely to be related to the
    a. respiratory system.
    b. cardiovascular system.

19. Genu varum is (circle all that apply)
    a. an expected finding in a young toddler.
    b. clubfoot.
    c. bowlegs.
    d. swayback.

20. Appropriate sleep for a toddler is
    a. 10 hours/night.
    b. 8 hours/night with a 2-hour nap.
    c. 11.5 hours/24 hours.
    d. whatever allows for rest.

21. Poor weight gain at any age in childhood is cause for concern. List four reasons for this _____ _____ _____ _____.

22. Impaired language development may be the result of (circle all that apply)
    a. hearing impairment.
    b. neglect.
    c. mental retardation.
    d. repeated bouts of otitis media.

23. Adolescents often have orthopedic problems. This can result from (circle all that apply)
    a. sports injuries.
    b. rapid growth spurts.
    c. poor coordination.
    d. immature judgments.
    e. extreme sports.

24. Depression among adolescents is more common than one would wish. If an adolescent admits to being depressed, the nurse should
    a. present cheerful suggestions.
    b. encourage the client to visit a school counselor.
    c. ask about the possibility of suicide.
    d. urge the child to become involved in school activities.

25. Reproductive assessment for an adolescent who is not sexually active should include (circle all that apply)
    a. a complete history of secondary sex characteristics and their appearance.
    b. questions about the client's expectations of physical development.
    c. assessment of the child's knowledge of menses, nocturnal emissions, etc.
    d. a pelvic exam for the female.
    e. a testicular exam for the male.
    f. a genital exam for the female.

CASE STUDY

You meet Angie as your client in a well-child clinic when she brings her 1-month-old infant in for a first exam. Angie is clearly in love with her little daughter Jadin, glowing with her praises, but also anxious about "some things." Jadin is breastfeeding and eats about every 1 to 2 hours. Angie is experiencing a little breast tenderness, but that is getting better daily. She is quite concerned that Jadin is getting enough milk, though she thinks she must be because she falls asleep contentedly after breastfeeding. Angie's concerns are as follows: She loves to watch her baby sleep but sometimes notices that Jadin breathes irregularly, with tiny spaces between breaths and then one or two little short gasps. She does say the baby exhibits no distress. Further, Angie notes that if a little hand or foot escapes from her blankets, the skin on her extremities takes on a mottled appearance. Angie also wonders if Jadin could be somewhat allergic to Angie's milk because she has tiny red lesions here and there on her face that appear more pronounced when she cries. She has noted too that Jadin seems to have some teeth coming in as she has noted what looks like two tiny white teeth in Jadin's gums.

- List the specific concerns for Jadin that Angie has indicated.

- As an introductory statement only, what can you tell Angie about the **probable** cause of the respiratory pattern, the skin lesions, the "teeth," and the mottled extremities?

- What specific assessment procedures would you do to discover if Angie's concerns are within normal limits or, indeed, signs of a problem?

- What is the minimum assessment protocol for a 1-month-old infant?

- What can you deduce about mother-infant bonding from the statements made by Angie? What behaviors can you be alert to that would give you additional information while you are with mother and baby?

- What nursing diagnoses would apply to Angie?
  What nursing diagnoses would apply to Jadin?

CLINICAL ACTIVITIES

Using the sample documentation form at the end of this chapter as a guideline, perform a history and physical assessment on a pediatric client. The following are considerations for selected age groups.

The Infant

Likely you will practice assessment of the infant with mannequin dolls, or you may have the opportunity to perform a newborn assessment in the nursery under the supervision of your instructor or an expert nursery nurse.

- Remember that hygiene is supremely important, and be sure to follow appropriately clean procedures for this assessment.
- At the same time, do not fail to implement Standard Precautions for your own protection from body fluids even of the newborn.

- If the exam is done in the presence of a parent, be sure to explain what you are doing and why you are doing it.
- Whenever appropriate, provide reassurance regarding your findings. An example might be, "I'm checking her for good muscle tone. Jadin has a brisk tone."
- Be careful to maintain warmth for the infant, exposing only what is necessary for a good assessment.
- Discuss the time frame and importance of the well baby visits with the parent.

The Toddler

- Planning for cooperation and fatigue is critical in the exam of the toddler. You will need the toddler's cooperation in order to assess developmental milestones, and so rapport is doubly important.

- If you cannot gain cooperation of the child, parent report of performance can be documented. For example, if there are no stairs in the assessment area, you will have to ask the parent how the child navigates stairs.
- After establishing some rapport, begin the assessment with those procedures that require the child's cooperation. Then if the child becomes tired or cranky, you can do those procedures such as cardiac auscultation that require minimal cooperation from the child.
- Be alert to signs of bonding and parent-child relationship during every encounter.
- As with the infant, discuss the time frame and the importance of continued well child visits.

The Adolescent

- Privacy and trust are critical with the adolescent.
- Derive as much of the history from the adolescent as possible. This is an opportunity to educate adolescent in the use of the healthcare system and the proper expectations he or she may have of a healthcare provider.
- Most of the physical assessment is no different from that of the adult. The history, however, should take into account the special risks, needs, and problems of the adolescent's development.
- Confidentiality is usually a critical issue with adolescents. You must be aware of the laws of majority in the state in which you practice and know what rights you are obliged to extend or withhold from an adolescent.
- The needs of a minor child can never be compromised in order to gain rapport. That is, the nurse can never promise secrecy over an issue that may be potentially harmful to the child. Seldom will a child withhold information in fear of exposure if the nurse gives reassurance that the decisions will be made for the protection of the child.
- Such statements as "I will only share information with your parent if I believe you are in harm's way" or "I will certainly give you the chance to share information with your parents in your own way" can be very helpful in gaining the adolescent's trust.

Note Appendices D and E in your textbook for reference in blood pressure norms for the various ages of boys and girls.

NURSING DIAGNOSIS

Look through the nursing diagnoses in Appendix A. How many of the nursing diagnoses relate directly to growth and development? This emphasis reflects the importance of considering growth and development norms while caring for clients of all ages.

Sample Documentation Form

Pediatric Assessment

Name: _____ Date: _____

Date of Birth: _____ Gestational age at birth: _____

Age: _____ Gender: _____

Focused analysis of current problem:

    Reason for visit: _____

_____

    Character: _____

    Onset: _____

    Duration: _____

    Location: _____

    Severity: _____

    Associated problems: _____

    Efforts to treat: _____

History

    Review of history related to pediatric measurements:

_____

    YES/NO   If YES, provide details:

Temperature

☐ ☐   Recent fever   _____

☐ ☐   Illness during past week   _____

☐ ☐   History of frequent illness or fever _____

Pulse

☐ ☐   Racing or irregular pulse   _____

☐ ☐   Cardiac disease   _____

☐ ☐   Tires easily with play   _____

Respirations

☐ ☐   Breathing difficulties   _____

☐ ☐   Shortness of breath   _____

☐ ☐   Cough or cold   _____

☐ ☐   Asthma or respiratory problems _____

☐ ☐   Allergies   _____

☐ ☐   Respiratory meds   _____

Growth and Development Concerns

☐ ☐   History of failure to thrive   _____

☐ ☐   Parent concern for child's growth _____

☐ ☐   Meets developmental landmarks _____

    Family history : _____

_____

Birth History *(for infants)*

    Gestational age: _____

    Complications of pregnancy: _____

    Complications of birthing (bleeding, medications, resuscitation): _____

    _____

    _____

    Apgar score (if available): _____

    Measurements (length, weight, head and chest circumference): _____

    _____

    Feeding (breast, bottle): _____

    Newborn assessment: _____

    _____

Medication history: _____

_____

Immunization history: _____

_____

Nutrition History

    Type and amount of foods eaten (variety, supplements): _____

    _____

    _____

    Eating skills (younger children: bottle, cup, chewing, utensil use; older children: eating patterns):

    _____

    _____

    Eating disorders: _____

    _____

Growth and Development Concerns

Yes	No	
☐	☐	History of failure to thrive _____
☐	☐	Parent concern for child's growth _____
☐	☐	Speech development _____
☐	☐	Motor development (creeping, walking, grasping, etc.) _____
☐	☐	School adaptation _____
☐	☐	Social skills for age _____
☐	☐	Family support _____
☐	☐	Safety (age-appropriate carriers, seat belts, protective devices) _____
☐	☐	Exposure to violence _____
☐	☐	Developmental landmarks met _____

For the Adolescent

    Safety (vehicles, sports, abuse): _____

    Social skills: _____

    Educational progress: _____

    Substance use or exposure: _____

    Sexuality (orientation, integration, knowledge, activity, molestation): _____

    _____

    Developmental landmarks (met/unmet): _____

Review of Systems (Age-Appropriate)

Allergies (note response): _____

Skin (lesions, care, and hygiene): _____

Head (injury, convulsions, headache, safety): _____

Eyes/vision: _____

Ears/hearing: _____

Neck, lymph: _____

Chest and lungs (asthma, allergies, infections): _____

Breast (development, drainage): _____

Heart and cardiovascular: _____

Abdomen (gastrointestinal, hernias, diabetes): _____

Musculoskeletal (development, injuries, sports, safety): _____

Neurologic (developmental landmarks, language): _____

Mental health (retardation, attention-deficit/hyperactivity disorder, depression, obsessive-compulsive disorder, anxiety): _____

_____

Genitourinary (number of wet diapers, pain, itching): _____

Reproductive (appropriate genitalia, sexual activity, menarche, circumcision, abuse, STD): _____

_____

Last Assessment Recorded

Date: _____

Record last assessment findings.

Temperature _____	Method _____	Height/length	_____
Pulse _____		Weight	_____
Respirations _____		**Infants:**	_____
Blood pressure _____		Head circumference	_____
BMI _____		Chest circumference	_____

Physical Assessment

Approach young children in order of procedures that require their cooperation, as they can become tired and/or uncooperative.

Vital Signs

		DATE OF ASSESSMENT			
Date					
Temperature	O = Oral A = Apical R = Rectal T = Tympanic				
Pulse	R = Radial A = Apical				
	Rhythm				
Respirations					
Blood Pressure Systolic / Diastolic					

Measurement for Young Children

	DATE OF ASSESSMENT			
Date				
Height or Length				
Weight kg lb				
BMI				
Evaluate until 1 year of age				
Circumference, Head (measure in cm)				
Head: Fontanels				
Circumference, Chest (measure in cm)				
Circumference, Abdomen (measure in cm)				

Also, plot the child's growth on one of the national standardized growth graphs. Consider standardized tools for assessment of development, such as the Denver Development II.

Please see text Chapter 25 for expected variations.

Skin (lesions, care, and hygiene): _____

Head (size, shape, fontanels [with infant], scalp, infestations, bruises): _____

_____

Eyes/vision (physical exam, red light reflex for infants, Snellen's, cover/uncover for older child): _____

_____

Ears/hearing (physical exam, placement, whisper, audiometry if available): _____

_____

Neck, lymph: _____

Chest and lungs: _____

Breast (development, drainage, BSE for adolescent): _____

_____

Heart and cardiovascular: _____

_____

Abdomen (hernias, organomegaly): _____

Musculoskeletal: _____

Neurologic (reflexes appropriate to age, developmental landmarks, language): _____

_____

Mental health (orientation, behavior): _____

_____

Reproductive/urinary (appropriate genitalia, vaginal discharge, urethral placement, descended testicles, signs of abuse, signs of STD, pregnancy): _____

_____

Analysis:

_____
_____
_____
_____

Nursing diagnoses: _____
_____

The Pregnant Female 26

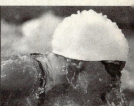

OVERVIEW

It is very important to keep in mind that pregnancy is not a medical condition, but the most natural and hopefully joyous of developments. Its expected course is precisely predictable and therefore directs the assessment and monitoring of the mother and the infant(s). With careful assessments, problems can often be addressed before outcomes are threatening. During the course of a pregnancy, there are many opportunities for teaching and support that can make significant differences to the health of the mother and infant(s).

You now have skills for the assessment of all body systems. Following are modifications and additions to assessment techniques that are required during pregnancy. Only those aspects of care that are unique to the pregnant mother and fetus are presented in this chapter.

ASSIGNMENT

CD-ROM content: Chapter 26
Companion wesite: www.prenhall.com/damico, Chapter 26

VOCABULARY EXERCISE

After completing the reading assignment, you should be able to define the **key terms** listed below. Refer back to the page number from the main text for help.

Amniotic fluid, 827
Areola, 827
Ballottement, 826
Braxton Hicks, 826
Chadwick's sign, 827
Colostrum, 828
Diastasis recti abdominis, 831
Dilation, 827
Ductus arteriosus, 825
Ductus venosus, 825
Effacement, 827
Embryo, 825
Fetoscope, 825
Foramen ovale, 825
Fundal height, 826
Fundus, 826
Gestational age, 825
Goodell's sign, 827
Hegar's sign, 826
Leopold's maneuvers, 854
Leukorrhea, 827

Lightening, 826
Linea nigra, 829
Mammary souffle, 829
McDonald's rule, 826
Menarche, 839
Montgomery's tubercles, 827
Mucous plug, 827
Multigravida, 826
Nägele's rule, 834
Physiologic anemia, 828
Pica, 824
Piskacek's sign, 826
Placenta, 824
Primigravida, 826
Quickening, 825
Ripening, 827
Striae gravidarum, 829
Supine hypotension syndrome, 829
Teratogen, 825
Viability, 825

ANATOMY EXERCISES

....

1. Label the bladder, the cervix, and rectum.

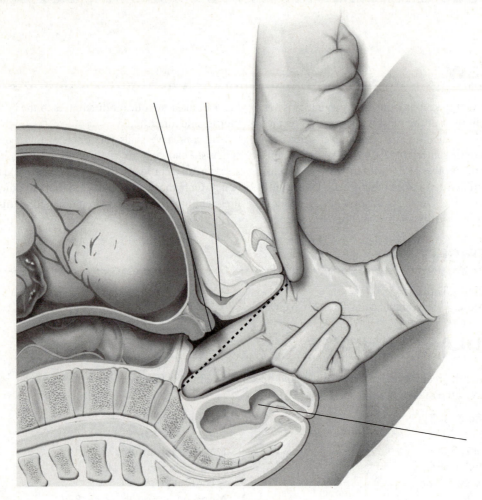

Figure 26–1

2. Given the proximity of the rectum and the vaginal canal, identify expected sensations during birth and dangers of contamination.

3. Given the location of the bladder and uterus, discuss the need to assess bladder content after birth.

STUDY FOCUS

. . . .

1. What are the major anthropometric measurements taken at the initial prenatal exam? Of what significance is the mother's body mass index at this time?

2. List the nutrients of special importance to a successful pregnancy.

3. Explain McDonald's rule and why it is an important assessment during pregnancy.

4. What changes to vital signs are expected in pregnancy?

5. Following are expected changes in skin physiology during pregnancy. Next to each one, indicate the assessment change you would look for.

    Increased pigment:

    Increased vascularity:

    Increased hair in growth phase:

6. Gastrointestinal changes during pregnancy result in several uncomfortable symptoms. Which of these symptoms has the potential to become a serious problem?

7. Serious urinary changes include increased susceptibility to infection. What assessment factors would alert the nurse to the existence of an infection?

8. What are the specific risks to a pregnancy from pre-existing hypertension?

9. What are the risks to mother and fetus from anemia?

10. When taking a medication history from a pregnant woman, how will the nurse know which medication may pose a risk to the fetus?

11. What is the focus of second-trimester teaching?

REVIEW QUESTIONS
....

1. Which of the following questions would be asked of a pregnant client during review of systems?
   a. What congenital anomalies are present in your family?
   b. What prescribed and over-the-counter medications do you use?
   c. When was your last menstrual period?
   d. What brings you in for care today?

2. An obstetrical history properly includes the following: last menstrual period, previous pregnancies, length of labor in pregnancies, complications in pregnancies, prepregnant medical conditions, size and weight of children born to this mother, EDC, gravida, and parity. This history is significant to
   a. future pregnancies.
   b. treatment of the newborn.
   c. the mother's reproductive health.
   d. anticipation of future medical conditions.
   e. all of the above.

3. The personal and social history of the pregnant woman should record her
   a. cultural and religious habits.
   b. exercise and recreation habits.
   c. work activities and exposures.
   d. opportunities for rest.
   e. all of the above.

4. An increase in pigment during pregnancy is responsible for
   a. part of the areolar changes.
   b. cutaneous tags.
   c. hair loss.
   d. chloasma.
   e. a and d.

5. Vital signs during normal pregnancy should reveal
   a. elevation of heart rate $10 \rightarrow 15$ beats per minute.
   b. elevation of respiratory rate (20 to 30%).
   c. drop in heart rate (10%).
   d. elevation of body temperature 2°F.

6. In cardiac auscultation of the pregnant woman, you find heart sounds exaggerated in volume. You are aware this is an outcome of
   a. increased blood volume of 30 to 40%.
   b. cardiac crisis secondary to increased oxygen demand.
   c. increased intra-abdominal pressure.

7. Nägele's rule is a straightforward mathematical formula for discovering the expected date of birth of an infant.
   a. true
   b. false

Matching: Indicate whether the following signs of pregnancy are positive (a) or presumptive (b).

8. fetal heart tones _____

9. amenorrhea _____

10. growth of abdominal size _____

11. sonogram of fetal parts _____

12. breast changes: increased size and nipple secretion _____

13. Goodell's sign _____

14. positive pregnancy test _____

15. Selected joints, fused in adults, become somewhat mobile in the second and third trimesters of pregnancy due to hormonal influence. Those joints are primarily (circle all that apply)
    a. thoracic vertebrae.
    b. hips.
    c. symphysis pubis.
    d. sacral-iliac/coccygeal.
    e. temporomandibular.

16. Mrs. Brown is Gr 4, P 5, ab 1, 5 LC. She has had
    a. four pregnancies, five live births, one abortion, and five living children.
    b. five pregnancies, one abortion, and four living children.
    c. four pregnancies, one set of triplets, and one abortion.
    d. five pregnancies, one elective abortion, and one set of twins.

Matching: Identify which of the following are physiologic (a) and which are abnormal (b) findings during pregnancy.

17. spontaneous bright red vaginal bleeding _____

18. elevation of systolic blood pressure _____

19. ankle edema relieved by foot elevation _____

20. persistent headache _____

21. urinary tract infection _____

22. proteinuria _____

23. During the first trimester a client presents with a hemoglobin of 11.5 g/dl. This value
    a. is above normal.
    b. indicates physiologic anemia of pregnancy.
    c. is an expected value at that time.
    d. cannot be judged without knowing the hematocrit.

24. What three specific findings on urinalysis would give cause for concern?

25. Blood loss above what level would be considered hemorrhage?

CASE STUDY

Lorraine, a 30-year-old gravida 4, para 3, is seen in the prenatal clinic for a routine appointment. As you take an updated history since her last appointment, she denies any "real problems." Picking up on her clue, you ask what she means by real problems. Lorraine tells you she is just tired of being pregnant. She has headaches a lot from not sleeping comfortably. She says she "is sick of having fat ankles and indigestion over every little thing." You are aware that she may well be tired of being pregnant. She may also have the warning signs of a very serious life-threatening problem.

- What assessments must you make initially?

- What findings on vital signs would be a red flag?

- How can you discriminate between dependent edema and edema?

- What laboratory tests should follow any negative findings on vital signs or edema assessment?

- Outline a focused assessment of a headache.

- What characteristics of a headache would you judge to be ominous for Lorraine during her pregnancy?

- What obstetrical history would be helpful to know at this point?

- What nursing diagnoses might apply to Lorraine?

CLINICAL ACTIVITIES

Using the sample documentation form as a guideline, take a complete history of a pregnant client or a lab partner able to role-play a pregnant client. If role-playing, decide before beginning what gravida and para the client will be so that an accurate history can be developed.

If working with a pregnant female, be sure to explain that you are learning to take histories and that there is no client reason for taking what will likely be an additional history. Pregnant women are justifiably concerned about the appearance of a complication, and may interpret your attention as the sign of a problem.

- Physical assessment of the pregnant client follows the same format as for the nonpregnant client in all systems except reproductive and abdominal.
- You will note expected changes and be alert for signs of complications.

- The physical assessment of the reproductive system and abdomen of a pregnant woman is not usually performed by a nurse without advanced training. As a practicing nurse you will, however, assist at this exam and also be available to answer questions your client may have.
- A calm, supportive manner is an asset to any caregiving and especially so for the pregnant client.
- As you perform your assessment, be sure to explain and reassure the client about procedures and findings. Use the guidelines offered at the end of this chapter.

As always, maintaining clean technique is essential, and protecting yourself from possible exposures is very important. Implement Standard Precautions as outlined in Appendices B and C of your textbook.

Sample Documentation Form

Assessment of the Pregnant Female

Name: _____ Date: _____

Age: _____ Marital Status/Significant Other: _____

Gravida: _____ Para: _____ AB: _____ Last Menstrual Period: _____ EDC: _____

Review of history of the pregnant female:

_____

YES/NO   If YES, provide details:
_____

Past Medical History

☐ ☐   Acute medical conditions   _____

☐ ☐   Chronic medical conditions   _____

☐ ☐   Gynecologic conditions   _____

☐ ☐   Gynecologic surgery   _____

☐ ☐   Infertility   _____

☐ ☐   Genetic conditions/concerns   _____

☐ ☐   Domestic abuse/violence   _____

☐ ☐   STD history   _____

☐ ☐   Nutrition history   _____

☐ ☐   Anemia   _____

☐ ☐   Cancer   _____

☐ ☐   Breast health (BSE)   _____

☐ ☐   Mental health   _____

Past Obstetric History

☐ ☐   Number of pregnancies   _____

☐ ☐   Number of term pregnancies   _____

☐ ☐   Abortions (type)   _____

☐ ☐   Deceased children (cause)   _____

☐ ☐   Obstetric complications   _____

               Prenatal   _____

               Intrapartal   _____

               Postpartum   _____

Current Health Status

☐ ☐   Acute medical conditions   _____

☐ ☐   Chronic medical conditions   _____

☐ ☐   Mental health conditions   _____

☐ ☐   Allergies   _____

☐ ☐   Medications   _____

                                         _____

                                         _____

☐ ☐   Infertility treatment   _____

☐ ☐   Gynecologic conditions   _____

☐ ☐   STD   _____

☐ ☐   Immunization status (hepB, hepA, influenza, tetanus, rubella) _____

☐ ☐   Sexual activity (number of partners) _____

                                         _____

☐ ☐   Smoking   _____

☐ ☐   Substance use   _____

☐ ☐   Abuse/violence   _____

☐ ☐   Nutrition   _____

☐ ☐   Nausea/vomiting   _____

☐ ☐   Vaginal bleeding   _____

☐ ☐   Urinary symptoms   _____

Family History

Medical history: _____

_____

Genetic implications: _____

_____

Social History

Support: _____

Employment: _____

Education: _____

Fitness activity: _____

Living arrangements: _____

Attitude toward infant: _____

Violence: _____

Review of history related to the current visit:

Focused symptom analysis of current problem:

Reason for visit: _____

_____

_____

Character: _____

Onset: _____

Duration: _____

Location: _____

Severity: _____

Associated problems: _____

Efforts to treat: _____

Physical Assessment:

Vital signs:

Blood pressure: _____ Pulse: _____ Temperature: _____ Respirations: _____

Height: _____ Weight: _____ BMI: _____

Pregnancy test: _____

Urine (note protein, red blood cells): _____

Hct/Hgb: _____

Blood type and Rh: _____

Fetal heart tones (location): _____

Skin: _____

HEENT: _____

Neck and thyroid: _____

Lungs: _____

Breasts: _____

Heart/cardiovascular: _____

_____

Gastrointestinal: _____

Neurologic (note reflexes): _____

_____

Musculoskeletal: _____

Extremities (note edema): _____

Abdomen (size, shape, fundal height, fetal heart tones, fetal movement): _____

_____

Pelvic Exam

External genitalia: _____

Pelvic measurements (if available): _____

Vagina: _____

Cervix: _____

Rectal exam: _____

Analysis:

_____

_____

_____

_____

Nursing diagnoses: _____

_____

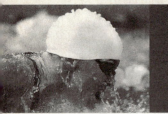

27 Assessing the Older Adult

OVERVIEW

You should now be able to assess all systems and regions of the body. Assessment of the older adult offers little to nothing new in techniques. Physical findings will be influenced by age and the presence of chronic health conditions. For example, some changes in skin that are expected in the older adult would be suspicious or even abnormal in a younger person. At the same time, the nurse must keep an open mind about expected behaviors. Some older adults are more active and more alert than their younger counterparts. Never allow the visual impact of an older adult to cause you to fail to ask appropriate questions or to test strength, range of motion, or cognitive function fully. Because hearing loss is quite pervasive, be sure that the client is given instructions he or she can hear clearly. It is quite easy for someone who simply misunderstands instructions or questions to appear to fail performance.

ASSIGNMENT

CD-ROM content: Chapter 27, especially clinical spotlight videos
Companion website: www.prenhall.com/damico, Chapter 27

VOCABULARY EXERCISE

After completing the reading assignment, you should be able to define the **key terms** listed below. Refer back to the page number from the main text for help.

Acrochordons, 900
Actinic keratoses, 900
Arcus senilis, 877
Cataract, 877
Cheilitis, 876
Cherry angiomas, 900
Lentigo senilis, 876
Mini–Mental State Examination, 881

Pinguecula, 877
Presbycusis, 877
Presbyopia, 877
Psychological distress, 881
Pterygium, 877
Seborrheic keratoses, 900
Senile purpura, 900
Xanthelasma, 876

STUDY FOCUS

1. Chapter 27 presents four theories of aging. Do any of these theories impact the assessment of the older adult in a specific way?

2. Even though older adults may be of desirable weight or above, they may have a gaunt face suggestive of underweight. What is responsible for this appearance? What risk factors are associated with this situation?

3. Due to decreased tone and peristalsis of the colon, certain undesirable gastrointestinal conditions become more common in the older adult. These are _____, _____, and _____.

4. What are the changes in aging that most affect eating and, consequently, nutrition?

5. Asking about depression or other mood disorders is important for the client of any age. What additional explanation might the nurse need to give for the older client to feel free to describe such problems?

6. People of all ages identify times when their memory fails. How would you help the client determine if memory problems are typical or may indicate neurologic changes?

7. What changes, if any, should be expected in the older adult's vital signs?

8. Though skin changes can be quite dramatic in the older person, bruises, scratches, and burns must be evaluated as possible signs of abuse. What questions can the nurse ask that might inspire an older client to reveal abuse?

9. What risks may follow if an older client has a loss of olfactory function?

10. Shortening of the spine is common in older adults. What are some possible findings that would accompany these changes?

REVIEW QUESTIONS

1. Assessment of the skin of the older adult may reveal (circle all that apply)
   a. lentigo.
   b. overgrowth of body hair.
   c. milia.
   d. cheilitis.
   e. excessive perspiration.

2. On identifying a loss of hearing in the older client, the appropriate nursing intervention would be
   a. referral for possible presbycusis.
   b. explanation to the client that some hearing loss is normal.
   c. examination of the ear canal for wax occlusion.
   d. referral for hearing assistance.

3. Standards for blood pressure for the older adult are
   a. unchanged.
   b. lower than for the middle adult.
   c. set higher for the older adult.

4. CDC recommendations for pneumococcal vaccination for the older adult are
   a. yearly in the fall.
   b. after age 65, then every 5 years.
   c. one time after age 65.

5. Dysphagia alone or with indigestion
   a. is an expected change with aging.
   b. is a possible sign of pathology.
   c. is usually related to an intemperate diet for age.
   d. can often promote poor nutrition.

6. Depressive symptoms are often accompanied by which of the following behaviors? (circle all that apply)
   a. poor nutrition
   b. increased alcohol intake
   c. social isolation
   d. poor hygiene

7. A decrease in the amount and quality of sleep at night in the older adult (circle all that apply)
   a. are to be expected.
   b. can be caused by poor exercise habits.
   c. can be a sign of depression.
   d. can be the result of increased napping.
   e. all of the above.

8. Sexual activity in the older adult
   a. can be more hazardous regarding STD.
   b. should be respected and supported.
   c. is a proper focus of the nurse providing holistic care.
   d. all of the above.

9. How do the risks of smoking by a 35-year-old differ from those of an 85-year-old?

10. Involving caregivers or family members in a health history for an older adult
    a. may improve upon the completeness and accuracy of an interview.
    b. must only be done with the permission of a client who is competent.
    c. may reveal inconsistencies in reports.
    d. may alert caregivers to concerns they had not yet identified.
    e. all of the above.

11. List the systems that may be partially evaluated by the prepared nurse on doing a general survey.

12. Identify the vessels the nurse would be sure to auscultate in the older adult. Does this differ from the younger adult? If so, how?

13. Adventitious findings more common on an exam of the eye of the older adult than that of a younger person include (circle all that apply)
    a. glaucoma.
    b. cataract.
    c. Horner's pupil.
    d. diminished red light reflex.
    e. refractive error.
    f. nearsightedness.
    g. farsightedness.

14. Breasts of the older client will be _____ than those of a younger client.
    a. more dense
    b. less dense

15. A menstrual history should be taken on every female
    a. until menopause is complete.
    b. of any age.
    c. until age 65.

16. All chronic diseases become more likely with increased age. Following are some of the most common diseases of old age. (Circle all that apply.)
    a. breast cancer
    b. hypertension
    c. diabetes
    d. osteoarthritis

CASE STUDY

Donald, age 72, is your surgical client scheduled for a knee replacement. In your preoperative history interview, Donald tells you that he is not worried about postoperative pain because the knee has been hurting him plenty and it can't be much worse. He goes on to say that he plays tennis three times a week and for the last year has taken enough aspirin and ibuprofen to raise the drug company's profits! He says he has had some prostatitis but that with medication it is manageable. He takes no other medications and tells you that he has been an active athlete all his life. He is single, and most of his social life revolves around tennis and tennis friends.

- What additional history will you pursue regarding his medications?

- What are your concerns about the aspirin and ibuprofen?

- What advantage does Donald's long history of physical exercise bring to the situation?

- What concerns do you have for Donald's social needs if tennis becomes impossible for him?

- Of what particular importance are Donald's vital signs at this time?

- What specific physical assessment procedures are necessary at this time to prepare realistically for his postoperative course?

- What actual or potential nursing diagnoses might apply to Donald?

CLINICAL ACTIVITIES

Using the sample documentation form at the end of the chapter as guideline, perform a complete history and physical assessment on an older adult.

- ▶ Note that it may be necessary to allow increased time.
- ▶ Though it is important to establish rapport, it is equally important to plan the assessment in such a way that tests that require maximum cognition and physical stamina be carried out before the client becomes fatigued.
- ▶ If you are dealing with a client who has limitations, plan to alter or supplement equipment before you begin.

For example, if the client has limited mobility, the usual examination table may not be an option. An armed chair and a bed may have to be substituted.

- ▶ Precautions for the nurse should not be compromised. Blood and body fluids remain a concern regardless of the age of the client involved.
- ▶ Care in body mechanics for the nurse is also necessary if the client needs assistance in turning, etc.

Sample Documentation Form

Assessment of the Older Adult

Name: _____ Date: _____

Marital Status: S _____   M _____   D _____   W _____

Age: _____ Gender: _____

Health History

General Health

Functional Assessment

   Dressing, grooming, and hygiene (describe difficulties, if any): _____

   _____

   _____

   Eating (obtaining/shopping, preparing, chewing, tasting): _____

   _____

   _____

   Sleep/rest patterns (difficulty getting/staying asleep, orthopnea, pain/stiffness): _____

   _____

   _____

   Mobility (limited walking, driving, needs assistance): _____

   _____

   _____

   Love and belongingness (spouse, sexuality, proximity of family, socialization opportunities):

   _____

   _____

   Medications (List medications; ask how client obtains medications; ask how client organizes dosage
   and administration): _____

   _____

   _____

   Immunization history (influenza, pneumonia): _____

   _____

   _____

   Nutrition history: _____

   _____

   _____

   Chronic illness (cancer, diabetes, Parkinson's, Alzheimer's): _____

   _____

   _____

Review of history related to the current visit:

  Focused symptom analysis of current problem:

   Reason for visit: _____

   _____

   Character: _____

   Onset: _____

   Duration: _____

   Location: _____

   Severity: _____

   Associated problems: _____

   Efforts to treat: _____

  Review of Systems (Age-Appropriate)

   Allergies (note response): _____

   Skin (lesions, care, hygiene): _____

   Head (injury, convulsions, headache, safety): _____

   Eyes/vision (glasses, cataracts or surgery, pain, itching, dryness): _____

   Ears/hearing (hearing difficulty, hearing aids): _____

   Neck, lymph (pain, stiffness, swollen nodes): _____

   Chest and lungs (chronic obstructive pulmonary disease, allergies, infections, pneumonia, influenza):

   _____

   Breast (BSE): _____

   _____

   Heart and cardiovascular: (symptoms, history or cardiac event, stroke, blood pressure history): _____

   _____

   Abdomen (gastrointestinal, hernias, constipation, rectal itching/bleeding): _____

   _____

   Musculoskeletal (arthritis, fall risk, injuries): _____

   _____

   Neurologic (gait, coordination, tremor, decreased sensation): _____

   _____

   Mental health (mental status, depression, grieving, loneliness): _____

   _____

   Genitourinary (incontinence, irritable bladder, pain, itching): _____

   Female reproductive (sexual activity, menopause, Pap, gravida, para): _____

   _____

   Male reproductive (sexual activity/satisfaction, prostatitis, testicular self-exam): _____

   _____

 Physical Exam

  Vital Signs

   Temperature   _____   Height   _____

   Pulse   _____   Weight   _____

   Respirations   _____   BMI   _____

   Blood pressure   (right) _____

                    (left) _____

General survey: _____

_____

Skin (lesions, care, hygiene, bruising, signs of abuse): _____

_____

Head (size, shape, hair/scalp, infestations, bruises): _____

_____

Eyes/vision (physical exam, Snellen's, Rosenbaum's, anterior chamber, funduscopic): _____

_____

Ears/hearing (physical exam, whisper, audiometry if available): _____

_____

Neck, lymph (ROM, nodes): _____

_____

Chest and lungs (thoracic movement, dyspnea, adventitious sounds): _____

_____

Breast (scars): _____

_____

Heart and cardiovascular (peripheral circulation, bruits, heart sounds): _____

_____

Abdomen (hernias, organomegaly): _____

_____

Musculoskeletal (joint morphology, spine): _____

_____

Neurologic (reflexes, language, tremor, coordination): _____

_____

Mental health (orientation, behavior, Mini-Mental State Examination, level of alertness): _____

_____

Female reproductive/urinary (pelvic, Pap, STD, prolapse): _____

_____

Male reproductive/urinary (hydrocele, lesions, hernia, discharge): _____

_____

Analysis: _____

_____

Nursing diagnoses: _____

_____

Answer Key

Chapter 1:
Health Assessment

1. c 2. all 3. c 4. c 5. a 6. S
7. S if reported, O if observed
8. O 9. S 10. S 11. S 12. e
13. a 14. d 15. a

Chapter 2:
Wellness and Health Promotion

1. b 2. b 3. d 4. c 5. e 6. d
7. a, b, c, d
8. level of knowledge
   sexual orientation
   sexual activity desire
9. In general, what is your mood
   on a given day?
   Do you ever feel sad without
   knowing why you feel that
   way?
   Can you get to sleep when you
   wish?
   Do you awaken before you
   want to and find it difficult
   to return to sleep?
   Has your appetite or eating
   pattern changed?
   Do you find you have less
   energy for friends or fun?
   Do you find yourself to be
   easily irritable?
10. In what sports do you
    engage?
    Do you wear protective gear for
    that sport?
    Are you properly conditioned
    for that sport?
    Do you eat and drink
    appropriately before and
    while engaged in your sport?
11. a, b, c, d
12. cancer
13. violence
14. obesity
15. access to care
16. obesity/cardiovascular disease
17. trauma
18. *Healthy People 2010* leading
    health indicators

Clark and Leveal model of
   prevention
Health belief model
Health promotion model
19. See National Center for
    Chronic Disease Prevention
    and Health Promotion Website
20. seven, eight if hepatitis A is
    included, 16 vaccines

Chapter 3:
Health Assessment Across the Life Span

1. general to specific, skilled
   specific
2. c 3. a 4. a 5. 3.5 6. c 7. a
8. e 9. e
10. continued use

Chapter 4:
Cultural Considerations

1. c
2. dress, utensils, art and tools
3. c 4. b 5. e 6. e 7. b
8. accuracy in receiving a message
   from the client
   accuracy in giving a message to
   a client
   confidentiality if using a
   translator

Chapter 5:
Psychosocial Assessment

1. e 2. b
3. What goals do you have for
   yourself?
   Who forms your support
   group?
   What is your position in your
   family?
   What are your roles?
   How do you cope with
   problems?
   What are your spiritual
   beliefs?
4. poor eye contact
   poor grooming

accomplishment below
   potential
hopelessness in a hopeful
   situation
excessive anger
poor problem solving
inability to focus on problem
   at hand
irrational behavior
5. Diabetes can (not will) lower
   self-esteem by allowing the
   client to perceive him/herself as
   ill and/or different from others.
   It can promote social isolation
   as clients need to make food
   and exercise choices different
   from others.
6. sexual behavior not accepted
   by the culture
   role selection not acceptable to
   the society
   dress unacceptable to the
   society
7. a, b, e
8. adequate memory for age
   appropriate attention span for
   age
   orientation to person, time,
   and place
9. a, b, c, d
10. e

Chapter 6:
Techniques and Equipment

1. a, b, c, d, e, f
2. b
3. Light palpation is gentle,
   shallow, and used to assess
   moisture, texture, temperature,
   or lesions of the skin. Moderate
   palpation is used to assess most
   other structures of the body;
   joints, muscles, and organs.
   Deep palpation is used to
   assess organs that lie deep
   within the body.
4. a 5. a
6. a
7. softness or loudness

low or high (number of vibrations)

length of time the sound persists

clear hollow, muffled or harsh
8. low-pitched sounds
9. privacy, warmth

Chapter 7:
General Survey

1. a, b, c, d
2. neurologic impairment, substance abuse, trauma, musculoskeletal deficit, weakness
3. c 4. e 5. a, b, c
6. less stable, less stable, as stable as compared to external influences
7. temporal, carotid, brachial, radial, femoral, popliteal, posterior tibial, dorsalis pedis arteries
8. b, d
9. time, location, rate, rhythm, amplitude, and bilateral symmetry
10. Repeat measurement to confirm.
11. cardiac output, blood volume, peripheral vascular resistance, blood viscosity, vessel compliance
12. low
13. to avoid the auscultatory gap
14. disappearance of sound, diastolic BP
15. brachial

Chapter 8: Pain Assessment

1. b
2. assessment, treatment, evaluation of treatment
3. b 4. b 5. b 6. b 7. b
8. a, b, c, d 9. b
10. BP, respiratory rate, pulse, and pupil size increased in early pain. Skin is pale and diaphoretic. These signs may be diminished or absent in chronic pain.
11. fear, anxiety, depression, lack of knowledge of source of pain, fatigue, lack of support, impact on activities of daily living, fear of pain control treatments

(e.g., fear of addiction or side effects of medications), believing pain is a punishment for client actions

Chapter 9:
Nutritional Assessment

1. diet history, physical assessment, anthropometric measurements, laboratory measurements
2. b 3. b 4. a
5. pregnancy, abdominal mass
6. B and C vitamins

Chapter 10:
The Health History

1. a 2. d 3. c 4. d 5. a 6. b
7. d 8. d 9. c 10. e 11. a
12. b 13. c 14. a 15. c 16. b
17. c

Chapter 11:
Skin, Hair, and Nails

1. b 2. d 3. b 4. a 5. e 6. a
7. b 8. b 9. c 10. b 11. b
12. d 13. c 14. c 15. d 16. e
17. e 18. c 19. b

Chapter 12: Head, Neck, and Related Lymphatics

1. e 2. a 3. e 4. e 5. c 6. a
7. b 8. c 9. b 10. e 11. c
12. e 13. a
14. facial CN VII
15. e
16. a, c, d, f, g
17. b, a, d, c or a, b, c, d
18. decrease in subcutaneous tissue altering slightly the client's face, thinning of hair on scalp, possible appearance of some hair on the female face, decreased muscle tone in neck
19. c 20. b 21. d 22. f 23. a
24. e
25. protective helmet/gear for occupational and hobby activities that could result in head injury, seat belt use in motor vehicles, attention to headache history, avoidance of intoxicants

Chapter 13: Eye

1. b 2. b 3. b 4. e 5. a 6. b
7. a 8. e 9. c 10. c 11. c
12. b 13. c 14. e 15. d 16. c
17. d 18. a 19. d 20. e 21. b
22. a 23. a 24. e 25. c

Chapter 14: Ears, Nose, Mouth, and Throat

1. b 2. a 3. c 4. b 5. a 6. e
7. d 8. b 9. a 10. c 11. a
12. a 13. a 14. a 15. b 16. e
17. d 18. b 19. b 20. c 21. b
22. e 23. e 24. b 25. a

Chapter 15:
Respiratory System

1. c 2. e 3. d 4. b 5. b 6. d
7. c 8. a 9. b 10. c 11. e
12. a 13. b 14. d 15. d 16. c
17. d 18. b 19. d 20. a 21. d

Chapter 16:
Breasts and Axillae

1. e 2. d 3. c 4. b 5. e 6. c
7. b 8. b 9. c 10. a 11. b
12. differences in underlying muscle mass side to side
13. b 14. a, b, c, e 15. d

Chapter 17:
Cardiovascular System

1. b 2. b 3. b 4. a 5. a 6. b
7. a 8. c 9. d 10. a 11. d
12. b 13. a 14. b 15. a 16. a
17. b, d, e, f, g
18. foramen ovale, ductus arteriosus
19. Splitting of S_2 will more likely be audible during inspiration.
20. cough, crackles, dyspnea, cyanosis, dizziness

Chapter 18: Peripheral Vascular System

1. b 2. a 3. b 4. b 5. a 6. c
7. c 8. a 9. a 10. b 11. a
12. b
13. a, b, d
14. at the elbow
15. arterial
16. tight Achilles tendon, strained calf muscle

17. posterior tibial and dorsalis pedis
18. a, b, d, e
19. blockage or defect in one side
20. pain, redness, swelling, heat over the area
21. d

Chapter 19: Abdomen

1. b 2. c 3. a 4. c 5. d 6. a
7. a 8. b 9. a 10. a 11. a
12. a, b, c, d, e 13. a 14. a 15. b
16. b 17. a 18. c 19. b 20. a
21. c 22. a 23. a 24. d 25. b

Chapter 20:
Urinary System

1. a 2. c 3. a 4. e 5. a, b, c
6. d
7. pain, burning, frequency, retention, abdominal pain
8. distended bladder, redness in urinary tissue, drainage, skin lesions in urinary tissue, odor to urine, color change to urine, concentration of urine, abnormal lab values (protein, RBCs, WBCs, increased specific gravity)
9. a, c, d 10. b 11. c 12. a
13. b 14. d 15. a 16. c 17. b

Chapter 21:
Male Reproductive System

1. c 2. c 3. e 4. e 5. a 6. d
7. a 8. b 9. b 10. c 11. c
12. a 13. b 14. a 15. b 16. a
17. d 18. b 19. b 20. d 21. b
22. a 23. b 24. b 25. c

Chapter 22:
Female Reproductive System

1. c 2. c 3. e 4. b 5. a 6. d
7. b 8. a 9. c 10. a 11. b
12. e 13. c 14. c 15. c 16. a

17. c 18. b 19. b 20. e 21. c
22. a, b, c, d, e, f 23. b 24. d
25. a 26. e

Chapter 23:
Musculoskeletal System

1. b 2. b 3. b 4. d 5. d 6. d
7. b 8. b 9. d 10. e 11. e
12. a 13. d 14. d 15. e 16. b
17. c
18. protein, calcium, vitamins C and D
19. steroids, thyroxin, heparin, diuretics, statins
20. pain, redness, swelling, deformity, asymmetry
21. b 22. b 23. a, c, e 24. a, e
25. fatigue, pain, client understanding of instructions

Chapter 24:
Neurologic System

1. e 2. b 3. c 4. d 5. b 6. b
7. a 8. e 9. d 10. c 11. b
12. c 13. d 14. d 15. e 16. b
17. c
18. areas of body involved, length of time involved, aura if any, level of alertness following, awareness of seizure by client, incontinence
19. diabetes, arthrosclerosis, syphilis, severe osteoporosis
20. b 21. a 22. c 23. b
24. a, b, c, d, e
25. hypertension, smoking, trauma, aneurysm

Chapter 25:
Assessment of Infants, Children, and Adolescents

1. c 2. a 3. c 4. a 5. b 6. d
7. e 8. c 9. a 10. c 11. b
12. b 13. a 14. b 15. b 16. a

17. c 18. a 19. a, c 20. c
21. neglect, renal disease, GI disease, endocrine disease, cardiovascular disease
22. a, b, c, d
23. a, b, c, d, e
24. c
25. a, b, c, e, f

Chapter 26:
The Pregnant Female

1. c 2. e 3. e 4. e 5. a 6. a
7. a 8. a 9. b 10. b 11. a
12. b 13. b 14. b 15. c, d
16. a 17. a 18. a 19. b 20. a
21. a 22. a 23. c
24. bacteria, protein, RBCs
25. 500 ml

Chapter 27:
Assessing the Older Adult

1. a, d 2. c 3. a 4. c 5. b
6. a, b, c, d
7. b, c, d
8. d
9. Both have a fire hazard. The older adult may have diminished sensation, increasing the risk of small burns leading to infections. Both have the potential for shortened life span related to pulmonary, cardiovascular, and oncological diseases.
10. e
11. musculoskeletal, skin, neurologic, head and neck, facies, mental status, mood, nutrition
12. temporal, carotid, abdominal aorta; no
13. a, b, d, g
14. b
15. b
16. a, b, c, d

D'Amico and Barbarito
Health History/Interview Checklist

Student _____   Date _____

Use the interview information provided in Chapter 10 to collect the following data.

Health History	Performance (S or U)*	Comments
Preinteraction Phase:		
Name		
Address		
Telephone		
Age		
Date of birth		
Birthplace		
Gender		
Marital status		
Race		
Religion		
Occupation		
Source of information		
Reliability of historian		
Present History/Illness:		
Reason for seeking care		
Health beliefs/practices		
Health patterns		
Medications		
Health goals		

(continued)

Health History/Interview Checklist *(continued)*

Health History	Performance (S or U)*	Comments
Past History:		
Family history		
Childhood illnesses		
Immunizations		
Medical illnesses		
Hospitalizations		
Surgery		
Injury		
Blood transfusions		
Emotional/psychiatric problems		
Allergies:		
Food		
Medications		
Environment		
Use of tobacco		
Use of alcohol		
Use of illicit drugs		

*Legend S–Satisfactory   U–Unsatisfactory

Signature of Evaluator _____

D'Amico and Barbarito
Skin, Hair, and Nails Checklist

Student _____   Date _____

Use the information provided in Chapter 11 to perform this Assessment of Skin, Hair, and Nails.

Skin, Hair, and Nails Assessment	Performance (S or U)*	Comments

Gather Equipment:
  Examination gown
  Examination drape
  Examination light
  Nonsterile gloves
  Centimeter ruler
  Magnifying glass
  Penlight
  Wood's light		

Perform hand hygiene		
Use standard precautions		
Provide for privacy		
Inspect the Skin: Position the client		
Instruct the client		
Observe for cleanliness and use the sense of smell to determine body odor		
Observe the skin tone		
Inspect the skin for even pigmentation over the body		
Inspect the skin for superficial arteries and veins		
Palpation of the Skin: Instruct the client		
Determine the skin temperature		

(continued)

Skin, Hair, and Nails Checklist *(continued)*

Skin, Hair, and Nails Assessment	Performance (S or U)*	Comments
Assess the amount of moisture on the skin surface		
Palpate the skin for texture		
Palpate the skin to determine its thickness		
Palpate the skin for elasticity		
Inspect and palpate the skin for lesions		
Palpate the skin for tenderness		
Inspect the Scalp and Hair: Instruct the client		
Observe for cleanliness		
Observe the hair color		
Assess the texture of the hair		
Observe the amount and distribution of the hair throughout the scalp		
Inspect the scalp for lesions		
Assessment of the Nails: Instruct the client		
Assess for hygiene		
Inspect the nails for an even, pink undertone		
Assess capillary refill		

Skin, Hair, and Nails Checklist *(continued)*

Skin, Hair, and Nails Assessment	Performance (S or U)*	Comments
Inspect and palpate the nails for shape and contour		
Palpate the nails to determine their thickness, regularity, and attachment to the nail bed		
Inspect and palpate the cuticles		
Perform hand hygiene		
Document findings		

*Legend S–Satisfactory   U–Unsatisfactory

Signature of Evaluator _____

D'AMICO AND BARBARITO
HEAD, NECK, AND RELATED LYMPHATICS CHECKLIST

Student _____   Date _____

Use the information provided in Chapter 12 to perform this Assessment of Head, Neck, and Lyphatics.

Head, Neck, and Lymphatics Assessment	Performance (S or U)*	Comments
Gather Equipment: Examination gloves Glass of water Stethoscope		
Perform hand hygiene		
Use standard precaution		
Provide for privacy		
Head: Position the client		
Instruct the client		
Inspect the head and scalp		
Inspect the face		
Observe movements of head, face, and eyes		
Assess cranial nerves III, IV, and VI		
Palpate the head and scalp		
Confirm skin and tissue integrity		
Palpate the temporal artery		
Auscultate the temporal artery		
Test the Range of Motion (ROM) of the Temporo Mandibular Joints (TMJ)		

Head, Neck, and Related Lymphatics Checklist *(continued)*

Head, Neck, and Lymphatics Assessment	Performance (S or U)*	Comments
Neck: Inspect the neck for skin color, integrity, shape, and symmetry		
Test ROM of the neck		
Observe the carotid arteries and jugular veins		
Palpate the trachea		
Inspect the thyroid gland		
Palpate the thyroid gland from behind the client		
Palpate the thyroid gland in front of client		
Auscultate the thyroid		
Palpate the lymph nodes of head and neck		
Perform hand hygiene		
Document findings		

*Legend S–Satisfactory   U–Unsatisfactory

Signature of Evaluator _____

D'AMICO AND BARBARITO
EYE CHECKLIST

Student _____   Date _____

Use the information provided in Chapter 13 to perform this Assessment of the Eyes.

Eye Assessment	Performance (S or U)*	Comments

Gather Equipment:
  Visual acuity charts
  Opaque card or eye cover
  Penlight
  Cotton-tipped applicator
  Ophthalmoscope
  Nonsterile gloves		

Perform hand hygiene		
Use standard precautions		
Provide for privacy		
Testing Visual Acuity: Distant Vision: Position the client		
Instruct the client		
Test distant vision		
Near Vision: Position the client		
Instruct the client		
Test near vision		
Test visual field by confrontation		
Test the six cardinal fields of gaze		
Assess the corneal light reflex		
Perform the cover test		
Inspect the pupils		

Eye Checklist *(continued)*

Eye Assessment	Performance (S or U)*	Comments
Test for accommodation of papillary response		
Evaluate papillary response		
Test the corneal light reflex		
Inspect the external eye		
Palpate the eye		
Examine the conjunctiva and sclera under the lower eyelid		
Inspect the fundus using the ophthalmoscope		
Perform hand hygiene		
Document findings		

*Legend S–Satisfactory   U–Unsatisfactory

Signature of Evaluator _____

D'Amico and Barbarito
Ears, Nose, Mouth, and Throat Checklist

Student _____   Date _____

Use the information provided in Chapter 14 to perform this Assessment of the Ears, Nose, Mouth, and Throat.

Ears, Nose, Mouth, and Throat Assessment	Performance (S or U)*	Comments
Gather Equipment: Examination gown Nonsterile gloves Otoscope Tuning fork Nasal speculum Penlight Gauze pads Tongue blade		
Perform hand hygiene		
Use standard precautions		
Provide for privacy		
Obtain history/assess hearing		
Ear: Position the client		
Instruct the client		
Inspect the external ear for symmetry, proportion, color, and integrity		
Palpate the auricle and push on the tragus		
Palpate the mastoid process lying directly behind the ear		
Inspect the auditory canal using the otoscope		
Examine the tympanic membrane using the otoscope		
Perform the whisper test		

Ears, Nose, Mouth, and Throat Checklist *(continued)*

Ears, Nose, Mouth, and Throat Assessment	Performance (S or U)*	Comments
Perform the Rinne test		
Perform the Weber test		
Perform the Romberg test		
Nose and Sinuses: Instruct the client		
Inspect the nose for shape, skin lesions, and signs of infection		
Test for patency		
Palpate the external nose for tenderness, swelling, and stability		
Inspect the nasal cavity using a nasal speculum		
Palpate the sinuses		
Percuss the sinuses		
Transilluminate the sinuses		
Mouth and Throat: Inspect and palpate the lips		
Inspect the teeth		
Inspect and palpate the buccal mucosa, gums, and tongue		
Inspect the salivary glands		
Inspect the throat		
Perform hand hygiene		
Document findings		

*Legend S–Satisfactory   U–Unsatisfactory

Signature of Evaluator _____

D'Amico and Barbarito
Respiratory System Checklist

Student _____   Date _____

Use the information provided in Chapter 15 to perform this Assessment of the Respiratory System.

Respiratory System Assessment	Performance (S or U)*	Comments

Gather Equipment:
  Examination gown and drape
  Nonsterile gloves
  Examination light
  Stethoscope
  Skin marker
  Metric ruler
  Tissues
  Face mask		

Perform hand hygiene		
Use standard precautions		
Provide for privacy		
Inspect the Anterior Thorax: Position the client		
Instruct the client		
Observe skin color		
Inspect the structures of the anterior thorax		
Inspect for symmetry		
Inspect chest configuration		
Count the respiratory rate		
Inspect the Lateral Thorax: Position the client		
Instruct the client		
Observe skin color		

Respiratory System Checklist *(continued)*

Respiratory System Assessment	Performance (S or U)*	Comments
Inspect the structure of the thorax		
Inspect for symmetry		
Inspect the Posterior Thorax: Instruct the client		
Observe skin color		
Inspect the structures of the posterior thorax		
Inspect for symmetry		
Observe respirations		
Palpation of the Posterior Thorax: Instruct the client		
Lightly palpate the posterior thorax		
Palpate and count ribs and intercostal spaces		
Palpate for respiratory expansion		
Palpate for tactile fremitus		
Percussion of the Posterior Thorax: Visualize the landmarks		
Recall the expected findings (resonance)		
Instruct the client		
Percuss the lungs		
Percuss for movement of diaphragmatic excursion		

(continued)

Respiratory System Checklist *(continued)*

Respiratory System Assessment	Performance (S or U)*	Comments
Auscultate the Posterior Thorax: Instruct the client		
Visualize the landmarks		
Auscultate for tracheal sounds		
Auscultate for bronchial sounds		
Auscultate for bronchovesicular sounds		
Auscultate for vesicular sounds		
Voice Sounds: Instruct the client		
Auscultate voice sounds, including bronchophony, egophony, and whispered pectoriloquy		
Palpation of the Anterior Thorax: Position the client		
Instruct the client		
Palpate the sternum, ribs, and intercostal spaces		
Lightly palpate the anterior thorax		
Palpate for respiratory expansion		
Palpate for tactile fremitus		
Percussion of the Anterior Thorax: Visualize the landmarks		

Respiratory System Checklist *(continued)*

Respiratory System Assessment	Performance (S or U)*	Comments
Recall the expected findings		
Instruct the client		
Percuss the lungs		
Auscultation of the Anterior Thorax: Instruct the client		
Auscultate the trachea		
Auscultate the apices		
Auscultate the bronchi		
Auscultate the lungs		
Interpret the findings		
Perform hand hygiene		
Document findings		

*Legend S–Satisfactory   U–Unsatisfactory

Signature of Evaluator _____

D'AMICO AND BARBARITO
BREAST AND AXILLAE CHECKLIST

Student _____   Date _____

Use the information provided in Chapter 16 to perform this Assessment of the Breast and Axillae System.

Breast and Axillae System Assessment	Performance (S or U)*	Comments

Gather Equipment:
  Examination gown and drape
  Nonsterile gloves
  Small pillow or rolled towel
  Metric ruler		

Perform hand hygiene		
Use standard precautions		
Provide for privacy		
Inspect the Breast: Position the client		
Instruct the client		
Inspect and compare size and symmetry of the breast		
Inspect for skin color		
Inspect for venous patterns		
Inspect for moles or other markings		
Inspect the areolae		
Inspect the nipples		
Observe the breast for shape, surface characteristics, and bilateral pull of suspensory ligaments		

Breast and Axillae System Checklist *(continued)*

Breast and Axillae System Assessment	Performance (S or U)*	Comments
Inspect with the client's arm over the head		
Inspect with the client's hand pressed against her waist		
Inspect with the client's hands pressed together at level of the waist		
Inspect the client leaning forward from waist		
Palpation of the Breast: Position the client		
Instruct the client		
Palpate skin texture		
Palpate the breast		
Palpate the nipple and areolae		
Examine the Axillae: Instruct the client		
Position the client		
Inspect the Male Breast: Position the client		
Instruct the client		
Inspect the male breast		
Palpation of the Male Breast: Position the client		
Instruct the client		
Palpate the male breast		

(continued)

Breast and Axillae System Checklist *(continued)*

Breast and Axillae System Assessment	Performance (S or U)*	Comments
Palpate the nipple		
Inspect the Male Axillae		
Perform hand hygiene		
Document findings		

*Legend S–Satisfactory   U–Unsatisfactory

Signature of Evaluator _____

D'AMICO AND BARBARITO
CARDIOVASCULAR SYSTEM CHECKLIST

Student _____   Date _____

Use the information provided in Chapter 17 to perform this Assessment of the Cardiovascular System.

Cardiovascular System Assessment	Performance (S or U)*	Comments

Gather Equipment:
  Examination gown
  Examination drape
  Stethoscope
  Metric ruler
  Doppler
  Lamp		

Provide hand hygiene		
Use standard precautions		
Provide for privacy		
Inspection: Position the client		
Instruct the client		
Inspect the face, lips, ears, and scalp		
Inspect the jugular veins		
Inspect the carotid arteries		
Inspect the hands and fingers		
Inspect the chest		
Inspect the abdomen		
Inspect the legs		
Inspect the skeletal structure		

(continued)

Cardiovascular System Checklist *(continued)*

Cardiovascular System Assessment	Performance (S or U)*	Comments
Palpation: Palpate the chest		
Palpate the carotid pulses		
Percussion: Percuss the chest to determine the cardiac border		
Auscultate: Auscultate the chest with the diaphragm of the stethoscope		
Auscultate the chest wall with the bell of the stethoscope		
Auscultate the carotid arteries		
Compare the apical pulse to a carotid pulse		
Repeat the auscultation of the chest in the left lateral and sitting positions		
Perform hand hygiene		
Document findings		

*Legend S–Satisfactory   U–Unsatisfactory

Signature of Evaluator _____

D'AMICO AND BARBARITO
PERIPHERAL VASCULAR SYSTEM CHECKLIST

Student _____   Date _____

Use the information provided in Chapter 18 to perform this Assessment of the Peripheral Vascular System.

Peripheral Vascular System Assessment	Performance (S or U)*	Comments

Gather Equipment:
  Examination gown
  Sphygmomanometer
  Stethoscope
  Doppler		

Perform hand hygiene		
Use standard precautions		
Provide for privacy		
Blood Pressure: Position the client		
Instruct the client		
Assist the client to a supine position		
Take the blood pressure in both arms		
Take the blood pressure in both legs		
Carotid Arteries: Inspect the neck for carotid pulsations		
Palpate the carotid pulses		
Auscultate the carotid pulses		
Arms: Inspect the hands		
Observe the capillary refill in both hands		

(continued)

Peripheral Vascular System Checklist *(continued)*

Peripheral Vascular System Assessment	Performance (S or U)*	Comments
Place both arms together and compare their sizes		
Palpate the radial pulse		
Palpate the brachial pulses		
Perform Allen's test		
Palpate the epitrochlear lymph node in each arm		
Palpate the axillary lymph nodes		
Legs: Inspect the legs		
Compare the sizes of both legs		
Palpate the legs for temperature		
Inspect the legs for the presence of superficial veins		
Perform the manual compression test		
Perform Trendelenburg's test		
Test for Homans' sign		
Palpate the inguinal lymph nodes		
Palpate both femoral pulses		
Palpate both popliteal pulses		
Palpate both dorsalis pedis pulses		

Peripheral Vascular System Checklist *(continued)*

Peripheral Vascular System Assessment	Performance (S or U)*	Comments
Palpate both posterior tibial pulses		
Assess for arterial supply to the lower legs and feet		
Test the lower legs for muscle strength		
Test the lower legs for sensation		
Check for edema of the legs		
Inspect the toenails for color and thickness		
Perform hand hygiene		
Document findings		

*Legend S–Satisfactory   U–Unsatisfactory

Signature of Evaluator _____

D'AMICO AND BARBARITO
ABDOMEN CHECKLIST

Student _____   Date _____

Use the information provided in Chapter 19 to perform this Assessment of the Abdomen.

Abdominal Assessment	Performance (S or U)*	Comments
Gather Equipment: 　Examination gown 　Examination drape 　Nonsterile gloves 　Examination light 　Stethoscope 　Skin marker 　Metric ruler 　Tissues 　Tape measure		
Perform hand hygiene		
Use standard precautions		
Provide for privacy		
Inspect the Abdomen: 　Position the client		
Instruct the client		
Determine the contour of the abdomen		
Observe the position of the umbilicus		
Observe skin color		
Observe the location and characteristics of lesions, scars, and abdominal markings		
Observe the abdomen for symmetry, bulging, or masses		
Observe the abdominal wall for movement		

Abdomen Checklist *(continued)*

Abdomen Assessment	Performance (S or U)*	Comments
Auscultation of the Abdomen: Instruct the client		
Auscultate for bowel sounds		
Auscultate for vascular britis		
Percussion of the Abdomen: Visualize the landmarks		
Instruct the client		
Percuss the abdomen		
Percussion of the Liver: Instruct the client		
Percuss the liver		
Percussion of the Spleen: Instruct the client		
Percuss the spleen		
Percussion of the Gastric Bubble: Instruct the client		
Percuss the gastric bubble		
Palpation of the Abdomen: Instruct the client		
Lightly palpate the abdomen		
Deeply palpate the abdomen		
Palpation of the Liver: Instruct the client		
Palpate the liver		

(continued)

Abdomen Checklist *(continued)*

Abdomen Assessment	Performance (S or U)*	Comments
Palpation of the Spleen: Instruct the client		
Palpate the spleen		
Additional Procedures: Palpate the aorta for pulsations		
Palpate for rebound tenderness		
Percuss the abdomen for ascites		
Test for psoas sign		
Test for Murphy's sign		
Perform hand hygiene		
Document findings		

*Legend S–Satisfactory   U–Unsatisfactory

Signature of Evaluator _____

D'Amico and Barbarito
Urinary System Checklist

Student _____   Date _____

Use the information provided in Chapter 20 to perform this Assessment of the Urinary System.

Urinary System Assessment	Performance (S or U)*	Comments

Gather Equipment:
  Examination gown
  Examination drape
  Nonsterile gloves
  Stethoscope
  Specimen container		

Perform hand hygiene		
Use standard precautions		
Provide for privacy		
Techniques and Normal Findings: Position the client		
Instruct the client		
Assess the general appearance		
Inspect the abdomen for color, contour, symmetry, and distention		
Auscultate the right and left renal arteries to assess circulatory sounds		
Kidneys and Flanks: Position the client		
Inspect the left and right costovertebral angles for color and symmetry		
Inspect the flanks for color and symmetry		

(continued)

Urinary System Checklist *(continued)*

Urinary System Assessment	Performance (S or U)*	Comments
Gently palpate the area over the left costovertebral angle		
Use blunt or indirect percussion to further assess the kidneys		
Left Kidney: Attempt to palpate the lower pole of the left kidney		
Attempt to capture the left kidney		
Right Kidney: Attempt to palpate the lower pole of the right kidney		
Attempt to capture the right kidney		
Urinary Bladder: Palpate the bladder to determine symmetry, location, size, and sensation		
Percuss the bladder to determine its location and degree of fullness		
Perform hand hygiene		
Document findings		

*Legend S–Satisfactory   U–Unsatisfactory

Signature of Evaluator _____

D'AMICO AND BARBARITO
MALE REPRODUCTIVE SYSTEM CHECKLIST

Student _____   Date _____

Use the information provided in Chapter 21 to perform this Assessment of the Male Reproductive System.

Male Reproductive System Assessment	Performance (S or U)*	Comments
Gather Equipment: Examination gown Examination drape Nonsterile gloves Examination light Flashlight Lubricant Slides and swabs to obtain a specimen of abnormal discharge		
Perform hand hygiene		
Use standard precautions		
Provide for privacy		
Inspection: Position the client		
Instruct the client		
Position yourself on a stool sitting in front of the client		
Inspect the pubic hair		
Inspect the penis		
Assess the position of the urinary meatus		
Inspect the scrotum		
Inspect the inguinal area		
Palpation: Palpate the penis		
Palpate the scrotum		

(continued)

Male Reproductive System Checklist *(continued)*

Male Reproductive System Assessment	Performance (S or U)*	Comments
Palpate the testes		
Palpate the epididymis		
Palpate the spermatic cord		
Palpate the inguinal region		
Palpate the inguinal lymph chain		
Inspect the perianal area		
Palpate the sacrococcygeal and perianal areas		
Inspect the anus		
Palpate the bulbourethral gland and the prostate gland		
Examine the stool		
Perform hand hygiene		
Document findings		

*Legend S–Satisfactory   U–Unsatisfactory

Signature of Evaluator _____

D'AMICO AND BARBARITO
FEMALE REPRODUCTIVE SYSTEM CHECKLIST

Student _____   Date _____

Use the information provided in Chapter 22 to perform this Assessment of the Female Reproductive System.

Female Reproductive System Assessment	Performance (S or U)*	Comments

Gather Equipment:
  Examination gown
  Examination drape
  Lubricant
  Pap smear equipment
  Speculum
  Handheld mirror		

Perform hand hygiene		
Use standard precautions		
Provide for privacy		
Inspect: Position the client		
Instruct the client		
Inspect the pubic hair		
Inspect the labia majora		
Inspect the labia minora		
Inspect the clitoris		
Inspect the urethral orifice		
Inspect the vaginal opening, perineum, and anal area		
Palpate: Palpate the vaginal walls		
Palpate the urethra and Skene's glands		
Palpate the Bartholin's gland		

(continued)

Female Reproductive System Checklist *(continued)*

Female Reproductive System Assessment	Performance (S or U)*	Comments
Inspection with a Speculum: Select a speculum		
Hold the speculum in your dominant hand		
Insert the speculum		
Visualize the cervix		
Obtain the Pap Smear and Gonorrhea Culture: Perform an endocervical swab		
Obtain a cervical scrape		
Obtain a vaginal pool sample		
Obtain a gonorrhea culture		
Remove the speculum		
Bimanual Palpation: Palpate the cervix		
Palpate the fornices		
Palpate the uterus		
Palpate the ovaries		
Perform the rectovaginal exam		
Examine the stool		
Perform hand hygiene		
Document findings		

*Legend S–Satisfactory   U–Unsatisfactory

Signature of Evaluator _____

D'AMICO AND BARBARITO
MUSCULOSKELETAL SYSTEM CHECKLIST

Student _____   Date _____

Use the information provided in Chapter 23 to perform this Assessment of the Musculoskeletal System.

Musculoskeletal System Assessment	Performance (S or U)*	Comments

Gather Equipment:
  Examination gown
  Nonsterile gloves
  Examination light
  Skin marking pen
  Goniometer
  Tape measure		

Perform hand hygiene		
Use standard precautions		
Provide for privacy		
Assessment of the Joints: Position the client		
Instruct the client		
Inspect the temporomandibular joint on both sides		
Palpate the temporomandibular joints		
Palpate the muscles of the jaw		
Test for range of motion of the temporomandibular joints		
Test for muscle strength and motor function of cranial nerve V		
Shoulders: With the client facing you, inspect both shoulders		

(continued)

Musculoskeletal System Checklist *(continued)*

Musculoskeletal System Assessment	Performance (S or U)*	Comments
Palpate the shoulders and surrounding structures		
Test the range of motion of the shoulders		
Test for strength of the shoulder muscles		
Elbows: Support the client's arm and inspect the lateral and medial aspects of the elbows		
Palpate the lateral and medial aspects of the elbows		
Palpate the lateral and medial aspects of the olecranon process		
Test the range of motion of each elbow		
Test for muscle strength		
Wrists and Hands: Inspect the wrists and dorsum of the hands, for size, shape, symmetry, and color		
Inspect the palms of the hands		
Palpate the wrist and hands for temperature and texture		
Palpate each joint of the wrist and hands		
Test the range of motion of the wrist		

Musculoskeletal System Checklist *(continued)*

Musculoskeletal System Assessment	Performance (S or U)*	Comments
Test the range of motion of the hands and fingers		
Test for muscle strength of the fingers		
Hips: Inspect the position of each hip and leg with the client in a supine position		
Palpate each hip joint and the upper thighs		
Test the range of motion of the hips		
Test for muscle strength of the hips		
Knees: Inspect the knees		
Inspect the quadricep muscle in the anterior thigh		
Palpate the knee		
Palpate the tibiofemoral joint		
Test for the bulge sign		
Perform ballottement		
Test the range of motion of each knee		
Test for muscle strength		
Inspect the knee while the client is standing		
Ankles and Feet: Inspect the ankles and feet with the client sitting, standing, and walking		

(continued)

Musculoskeletal System Checklist *(continued)*

Musculoskeletal System Assessment	Performance (S or U)*	Comments
Palpate the ankles		
Palpate the length of the calcaneal (Achilles) tendon at the posterior ankle		
Palpate the metatarsophalangeal joints just below the ball of the foot		
Deeply palpate each metatarsophalangeal joint		
Test the range of motion of the ankles and feet		
Test for muscle strength of the ankles		
Test for muscle strength of the feet		
Palpate each interphalangeal joint		
Spine: Inspect the spine		
Palpate each vertebral process with your thumb		
Palpate the muscles on both sides of the neck and back		
Test the range of motion of the cervical spine		
Test the range of motion of the thoracic and spine		
Perform hand hygiene		
Document findings		

*Legend S–Satisfactory   U–Unsatisfactory

Signature of Evaluator _____

D'AMICO AND BARBARITO
NEUROLOGIC SYSTEM CHECKLIST

Student _____   Date _____

Use the information provided in Chapter 24 to perform this Assessment of the Neurologic System.

Neurological System Assessment	Performance (S or U)*	Comments

Gather Equipment:
  Examination gown
  Nonsterile gloves
  Percussion hammer
  Tuning fork
  Sterile cotton balls
  Penlight
  Ophthalmoscope
  Stethoscope
  Sterile needle
  Tongue blade
  Applicator
  Hot and cold water in
    test tubes
  Objects to touch, such as
    coins, paper clips, or
    safety pins
  Substances to smell, for
    example, vanilla, mint,
    and coffee
  Substance to taste such
    as sugar, salt, and lemon		

Perform hand hygiene		
Use standard precautions		
Provide for privacy		
Mental Status: Position the client		
Instruct the client		
Observe the client		
Note speech and language abilities		
Assess sensorium		

(continued)

Neurological System Checklist *(continued)*

Neurologic System Assessment	Performance (S or U)*	Comments
Assess memory		
Assess ability to calculate problems		
Assess ability to think abstractly		
Assess mood and emotional state		
Assess perception and thought processes		
Assess ability to make judgments		
Cranial Nerves: Instruct the client		
Test the olfactory nerve (cranial nerve I)		
Test the optic nerve (cranial nerve II)		
Test the oculomotor, trochlear, and abducens nerves (cranial nerves III, IV, and VI)		
Test the trigeminal nerve (cranial nerve V)		
Test the facial nerve (cranial nerve VIII)		
Test for vestibulocochlear (cranial nerve VII)		
Test the glossopharyngeal and vagus nerves (cranial nerves IX and X)		
Test the accessory nerve (cranial nerve XI)		

Neurological System Checklist *(continued)*

Neurologic System Assessment	Performance (S or U)*	Comments
Test the hypoglossal (cranial nerve XII)		
Motor Function/Cerebellar Function: Assess gait and balance		
Perform Romberg's test		
Perform the finger-to-nose test		
Assess ability to perform a rapid alternating action		
Ask the client to perform the heel-to-shin test		
Sensory Function: Assess ability to identify light touch		
Assess ability to distinguish the difference between sharp and dull		
Assess ability to distinguish temperature		
Assess ability to feel vibrations		
Test stereognosis, the ability to identify an object without seeing it		
Test graphesthesia, the ability to perceive writing on the skin		
Assess ability to discriminate between two points		

(continued)

Neurological System Checklist *(continued)*

Neurologic System Assessment	Performance (S or U)*	Comments
Assess point localization—the ability to identify an area of the body that has been touched		
Assess position sense of joint movement		
Reflexes: Assess the biceps reflex		
Assess the triceps reflex		
Assess the brachioradialis reflex		
Assess the patellar reflex		
Assess the Achilles tendon reflex		
Assess the abdominal reflexes		
Carotid auscultation		
Meningeal assessment		
Use of Glasgow Coma Scale		
Perform hand hygiene		
Document findings		

*Legend S–Satisfactory   U–Unsatisfactory

Signature of Evaluator _____

D'Amico and Barbarito
Assessment of Infants, Children, and Adolescents

Student _____   Date _____

Use the information provided in Chapter 25 to perform this Assessment of Infants, Children, and Adolescents.

Assessment of Infants, Children, and Adolescents	Performance (S or U)*	Comments
Gather Equipment: Examination gown Examination drape Stethoscope Sphygmomanometer Measuring tape Nonsterile gloves Ophthalmoscope with pneumatic bulb Appropriate-sized specula Tongue depressor Reflex hammer		
Perform hand hygiene		
Use standard precautions		
Provide for privacy		
Growth and Development: Obtain accurate height and weight		
Measure head circumference for children less than two years old		
Skin, Hair, and Nails: Inspect the skin for color and the presence of lesions, birthmarks, or discolorations		
Inspect the hair and nails for texture, distribution, and moisture		
Head and Neck: Inspect and palpate the skull for the presence of deformity		

(continued)

Assessment of Infants, Children, and Adolscents *(continued)*

Assessment of Infants, Children, and Adolescents	Performance (S or U)*	Comments
Palpate the lymph nodes of the head and neck		
Eyes and Vision: Inspect the eyes for symmetry, position, and movement		
Assess the inner eye structures		
Assess vision		
Ears and Hearing: Assess the outer ear		
Inspect the auditory canal and tympanic membrane		
Assess hearing		
Nose and Sinuses: Assess the nose for nasal patency and septal deviation		
Assess the sinuses		
Mouth and Throat: Assess the mouth and teeth		
Assess the pharynx and tonsils		
Chest and Lungs: Inspect the chest		
Auscultate the chest		
Cardiovascular: Assess the child for cyanosis and chest pulsations and determine the apical impulse		
Palpate pulse for symmetry, rate, and rhythm		

Assessment of Infants, Children, and Adolscents *(continued)*

Assessment of Infants, Children, and Adolescents	Performance (S or U)*	Comments
Auscultate heart sounds		
Abdomen:		
Inspect the abdominal contour and movement		
Auscultate the abdomen		
Palpate the abdomen		
Genitalia: Inspect the external genitalia		
Palpate the external genitalia		
Palpate the scrotum in males		
Musculoskeletal: Observe gait and movement		
Assess the upper extremities and neck		
Assess the lower extremities		
Assess the hips		
Assess the spine		
Neurological: Assess mental status		
Assess development and determine the presence of the infant reflexes		
Assess cranial nerve functioning and deep tendon reflexes		

(continued)

Assessment of Infants, Children, and Adolscents *(continued)*

Assessment of Infants, Children, and Adolescents	Performance (S or U)*	Comments
Assess for coordination, sensation, and movement		
Perform hand hygiene		
Document findings		

*Legend S–Satisfactory   U–Unsatisfactory

Signature of Evaluator _____

D'Amico and Barbarito
The Pregnant Female Checklist

Student _____   Date _____

Use the information provided in Chapter 26 to perform this Assessment of the Pregnant Female.

Assessment of the Pregnant Female	Performance (S or U)*	Comments

Gather Equipment:
   Examination gown
   Examination drape
   Sphymomanometer
   Adjustable light source
   Stethoscope
   Centimeter tape measure
   Reflex hammer
   Fetoscope or fetal doppler
   Ultrasonic gel
 Vaginal speculum
   Urine collection
     containers
   Urine testing strips
   Perineal cleansing wipes
   Otoscope and specula
   Tongue depressor		

Perform hand hygiene		
Use standard precautions		
Provide for privacy		

Pelvic Exam Equipment:
   Nonsterile gloves
   Labeled slides and
     fixatives or labeled
     containers for cytology
   Slide for vaginitis check
   Potassium hydroxide
   Saline drops
   Plastic or metal speculum
   Spatula		

Cytology brush or cervical broom Tissues Hand mirrors Water soluble lubricant Cervical culture swabs		

(continued)

Assessment of the Pregnant Female Checklist *(continued)*

Assessment of the Pregnant Female	Performance (S or U)*	Comments
General Survey: Measure the client's height and weight		
Assess general appearance and general mental status		
Take vital signs		
Test urine for glucose and protein		
Observe posture		
Skin, Hair, and Nails: Observe the skin, hair, and nails for changes associated with pregnancy		
Head and Neck: Inspect and palpate the neck		
Eyes, Ears, Nose, Mouth, and Throat: Inspect the eyes and ears		
Inspect the nose		
Inspect the mouth		
Inspect the throat		
Thorax and Lungs: Inspect, palpate, percuss, and auscultate the lungs		
Heart: Auscultate the heart		
Position the client		
Breast and Axillae: Inspect the breast		
Palpate the breast and axillae		

Assessment of the Pregnant Female Checklist *(continued)*

Assessment of the Pregnant Female	Performance (S or U)*	Comments
Extremities: Inspect and palpate the extremities		
Neurological System: Percuss the deep tendon reflexes		
Abdomen and Fetal Assessment: Inspect and palpate the abdomen		
Assess fetal growth through fundal height assessment		
Assess fetal activity		
Assess fetal lie, presentation, and position		
Auscultate fetal heart rate		
Assist the client into a lithotomy position		
External Genitalia: Inspect the external genitalia		
Palpate Bartholin's gland, urethra, and Skene's glands		
Inspect Vagina and Cervix: Observe the vagina		
Visualize the cervix		
Inspect the cervix		
Obtain a Pap smear and cervical cultures		
Proceed to pelvic assessment		

(continued)

Assessment of the Pregnant Female Checklist *(continued)*

Assessment of The Pregnant Female	Performance (S or U)*	Comments
Palpation of Pelvis: Assess the angle of the pubic arch		
Lubricate the gloved fingers		
Estimate the angle of the subpubic arch		
Assess the interspinous diameter		
Assess the curvature of the sacrum		
Measure the diagonal conjugate		
Palpation of Cervix, Uterus, Adnexa, and Vagina: Assess the cervix		
Perform bimanual palpation of the uterus		
Palpate the adnexa		
Assess vaginal tone		
Anus and Rectum: Perform the rectovaginal exam		
Measure the intertuberous diameter of the pelvic outlet		
Inspect the rectum		
Perform hand hygiene		
Document findings		

*Legend S–Satisfactory   U–Unsatisfactory

Signature of Evaluator _____

D'Amico and Barbarito
Assessing the Older Adult Checklist

Student _____ Date _____

Use the information provided in Chapter 27 to perform this Assessment of the Older Adult.

Assessment of the Older Adult	Performance (S or U)*	Comments

Gather Equipment:
  Examination gown
  Examination drape
  Examination light
  Penlight
  Stethoscope
  Ophthalmoscope
  Otoscope
  Substances to taste and
    smell
  Sphygmomanometer
  Centimeter measuring
    device
  Tongue depressor
  Cotton
  Vision screener
  Tuning fork
  Reflex hammer
  Sharp and dull objects		

Perform hand hygiene		
Use standard precautions		
Provide for privacy		
General Survey: Position the client		
Observe the client		
Evaluate nutritional status		
Take the vital signs		
Integumentary System: Inspect the skin for color		
Palpate the skin		

(continued)

Assessing the Older Adult *(continued)*

Assessment of the Older Adult	Performance (S or U)*	Comments
Measure and describe all skin lesions		
Inspect the hair		
Inspect the nails and nail beds		
Head and Neck: Observe the face		
Inspect the nose and nares		
Evaluate sense of smell		
Inspect the oral mucous membranes, gums, throat, and tongue		
Palpate and auscultate the carotid arteries		
Inspect and palpate the neck veins		
Evaluate the range of motion of the neck		
Eye: Inspect the eyelids, cornea, and iris		
Check the pupils for size, equality, and reactivity		
Measure visual acuity		
Check peripheral field of vision		
Inspect the fundus of the eye with an opthalmoscope		
Gently palpate the eyeball		

Assessing the Older Adult *(continued)*

Assessment of the Older Adult	Performance (S or U)*	Comments
Ear: Inspect the outer ear, ear canal, and tympanic membrane		
Evaluate hearing		
Respiratory System: Inspect the shape of the thorax		
Assess the chest walls and ribs		
Percuss the lung fields		
Auscultate the lung fields		
Breasts: Assess the female and male breasts		
Cardiovascular System: Auscultate the precordium		
Take the apical pulse		
Abdomen: Inspect the abdomen		
Auscultate the abdomen		
Percuss the abdomen		
Palpate the abdomen		
Genitourinary System: Female:		
Check the underclothing for staining		
Inspect the external genitals		
Perform a pelvic examination		

(continued)

Assessing the Older Adult *(continued)*

Assessment of the Older Adult	Performance (S or U)*	Comments
Examine the rectum		
Male: Check the underclothing for staining		
Inspect the external genitals		
Perform a rectal exam		
Musculoskeletal System: Position the client		
Assess the spinal column		
Assess all joints		
Assess the muscles		
Assess the feet		
Neurological System: Evaluate mental status		
Assess cranial nerves		
Evaluate balance and coordination		
Inspect for tremors of the head, face, and extremities		
Evaluate motor strength		
Evaluate sensation		
Evaluate reflexes with a reflex hammer		
Evaluate sleep sufficiency		
Perform hand hygiene		
Document findings		

*Legend S–Satisfactory   U–Unsatisfactory

Signature of Evaluator _____